Parsha ai

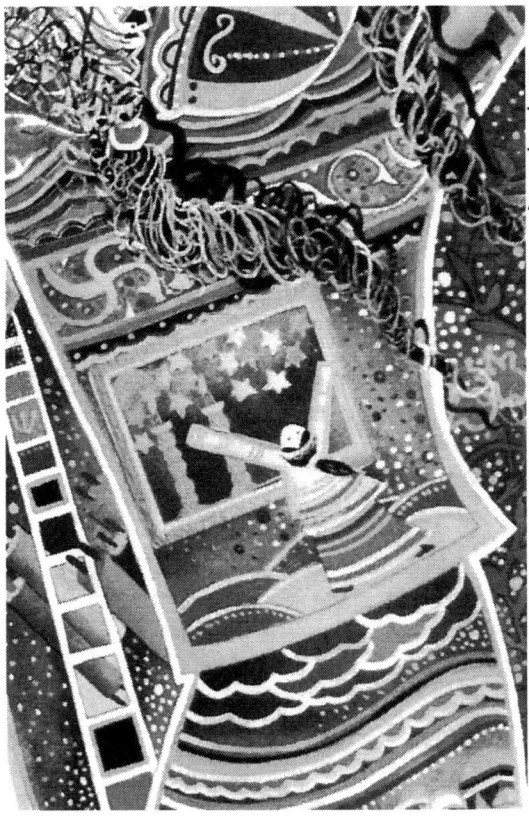

LIFE LESSONS FROM TORAH THROUGH THE STUDY OF THE PARSHA OF THE WEEK AND YOGA

PARSHA AND YOGA
Lessons from the weekly parsha and yoga

LINDA HOFFMAN

Copyright © 2014 Linda Hoffman

All rights reserved. No part of this publication may be reproduced, stored in a retrieval system, or transmitted in any form or by any means, electronic, mechanical, recording or otherwise, without the prior written permission of the author.

Linda Hoffman
www.parshaandyoga.com

DISCLAIMER

This book details the author's personal experiences with and opinions about yoga, Torah and personal characteristics. The author is not a healthcare provider.

The author and publisher are providing this book and its contents on an "as is" basis for informational purposes only and make no representations or warranties of any kind with respect to this book or its contents. The author and publisher disclaim all such representations and warranties, including for example warranties of merchantability and healthcare for a particular purpose. In addition, the author and publisher do not represent or warrant that the information accessible via this book is accurate, complete or current.

Users of said information and material, (1) voluntarily assume all risk related to said use, (2) waive all claims against author and publisher, and (3) agree to indemnify and hold author and publisher harmless.

The statements made about products and services have not been evaluated by the U.S. Food and Drug Administration. They are not intended to diagnose, treat, cure, or prevent any condition or disease. Please consult with your own physician or healthcare specialist regarding the suggestions and recommendations made in this book.

Except as specifically stated in this book, neither the author or publisher, nor any authors, contributors, or other representatives will be liable for damages arising out of or in connection with the use of this book. This is a comprehensive limitation of liability that applies to all damages of any kind, including (without limitation) compensatory; direct, indirect or consequential damages; loss of data, income or profit; loss of or damage to property and claims of third parties.

You understand that this book is not intended as a substitute for consultation with a licensed healthcare practitioner, such as your physician. Before you begin any healthcare program, or change your lifestyle in any way, you will consult your physician or other licensed healthcare practitioner to ensure that you are in good health and that the examples contained in this book will not harm you.

This book provides content related to topics of physical and/or mental health issues. As such, use of this book implies your acceptance of this disclaimer.

Acknowledgments

I could not have done this alone.

Over the years I have studied with many rabbis, rebbitzins and men and women like myself who brought Torah into their daily lives. Thank you for letting me join your classes and helping me to develop my understanding of Torah.

Thank you to my many yoga instructors.

Thank you to the wonderful team at Elance.com

Hanna, you are a wonderful editor. You knew where I was going and you grabbed hold of my hand and took me there.
Hanna Geshelin
Editing by Geshelin

Raphael Abecassis has graciously permitted me to use his artwork for the cover and inside sections. It is a segment from the beautiful "Eishes Chayil" embossed lithograph which graces my living room. Raphael Abecassis was born in Marrakesh, Morocco, in 1953, grew up in the south of Israel and is now living and painting in Natanya. He studied art at the College of Education in Beersheva.

Thank you, Hashem. I worked hard to use the potential you gave me. I am grateful.

Table of Contents

Parsha and Yoga ix

Book I
Bereishis/Genesis 3

    Bereishis (in the beginning) 5
    Yoga—Basic seated pose 9
    Noah (rest or comfort) 11
    Yoga–Cobbler position 15
    Lech Lecha (go for yourself) 17
    Yoga–Easy seated waist turn 21
    Vayeira (and he appeared) 23
    Yoga—Deeper seated twist 27
    Chayei Sarah (life of Sarah) 29
    Yoga—Downward dog in small steps 32
    Toldos (generations) 33
    Yoga—Your yoga workout is yours 36
    Vayeitzei (and he went out) 39
    Yoga—Resting pose for pause and peace 42
    Vayishlach (and he sent) 43
    Yoga—Warrior pose arms out 46
    Vayeishev (and he settled) 47
    Yoga—Child's pose for all Jacob's children 50
    Mikeitz (and in the end) 51
    Yoga—Standing plank pose 54

Vayigash (and he drew near)..55

Yoga—Mountain pose 58

Vayechi (and he lived) 59

Yoga—Bridge 62

Book II
Shemos/Exodus

63

Shemos (names)...65

Yoga—Mountain pose, swan dive, deep forward bend............67

Vaeira (and I appeared)..69

Yoga—Shoulder stand and plow 72

Bo (enter)..73

Yoga—Balance pose 76

Bishalach (when he let go)..77

Yoga—Patience..80

Yisro (abundance)...81

Yoga—Tree pose, scales of justice 83

Mishpatim (judgments)...85

Yoga—Find a yoga routine...89

Terumah (offering)...91

Yoga—A special place to do yoga 94

Tetzaveh (you shall command)......................................95

Yoga—Facial exercises, yoga clothing 97

Ki Sisa (when you elevate) 99

Yoga—Hold a position, knees to chest 102

Vayakhel (and he assembled) Pekudi (accountings of).........103

Yoga—Pick your yoga 106

Book III
Vayikra/Leviticus

109

Vayikra (and he called) 111

- Yoga—Pigeon pose 114
- Tzav (Command) 115
- Yoga—Deep breathing 117
- Shemini (Eighth) 119
- Yoga—Get ready for yoga 122
- Tazria (she bears seed) Metzora (infected one) 123
- Yoga—Back bend and forward bend 126
- Acharei (after the death) Kedoshim (Holy ones) 127
- Yoga—Concentration 131
- Emor (say) 133
- Yoga—Warrior success pose 137
- Behar (on the Mount) Bechukotal (in My Statutes) ... 139
- Yoga–Discipline 141

Book IV
Bamidbar/Numbers
....
143

- Bamidbar (in the desert) 145
- Yoga—Body placement, triangle pose 148
- Nasso (elevate) 149
- Yoga—Each day different 151
- Beha'alosecha (in your making go up) 153
- Yoga—Eagle 157
- Shelach (send for yourself) 159
- Yoga—Strongest warrior 163
- Korach (bald) 165
- Yoga—Pyramid 167
- Chukas (ordinance of) 169
- Yoga—Transition 172
- Balak (The Destroyer) 173
- Yoga—Donkey 177
- Pinchas (dark-skinned) 179

Yoga—Camel..182
  Mattos (tribes) Masei (journeys of) 183
  Yoga–Walk...188

Book V
Devarim/Deuteronomy

189

  Devarim (words)..191
  Yoga—Sore feet 193
  Va'eschanan (And I besought)...................................195
  Yoga—Protect and enhance.......................................198
  Eikev (this word means because and also means heel) 199
  Yoga—Chair pose 202
  Re'eh (see; before you) 203
  Yoga—Happy baby 207
  Shoftim (judges)...209
  Yoga—Plank pose...213
  Ki Seitzei (when you go out) 215
  Yoga—Core strength 217
  Ki Savo (when you come in)......................................219
  Yoga—Warnings and benefits 221
  Nitzavim (are standing) Vayeilech (and went).........223
  Yoga—Come back to exercise 227
  Haazinu (give ear) Vezos HaBerachah (and this is the blessing)229
  Yoga—Basic seated pose 233

References

235

Parsha and Yoga

What is Torah?
Torah, Judaism's most important text, is a deep and meaningful book that is applicable to all cultures and all times. Torah is the Hebrew Bible, the Old Testament, and known as the Five Books of Moses. The five books are Bereishis/Genesis, Shemos/Exodus, Vayikra/Leviticus, Bamidbar/Numbers, and Devarim/Deuteronomy. The Hebrew name is first and the English name follows. Each book of Torah consists of weekly parshas.

Torah is the story of the Jewish people from the creation of all things until the death of Moses. In Torah you find science, history, philosophy, ritual, ethics, stories of individuals and families, wars, slavery and more. All phases of human life are represented in Torah. It is a living Torah, relevant today to our lives and relationships, as much as it was when given at Mount Sinai. Torah is the foundation of ethics and morals for most cultures in the world.

Torah is written on a parchment scroll. Parchment is a thin material made from the split hide of a calf, sheep or goat. The scroll is then wound around two wooden poles. This is called a "Sefer Torah" and it is handwritten by a scribe who copies the text 100% accurately and then has it proofread by another trained scribe. There is no margin of error. These words are the same Torah words that were given to Moses. Wherever in the world you go, whatever synagogue you visit, every Torah is exactly the same. If a Torah gets damaged, or a letter rubs off, it is no longer "kosher" and must be fixed or replaced.

In modern printed form, a book, the Torah is usually called a "Chumash", which comes from the Hebrew word for the number five. My primary source for my weekly parsha reading is the Stone Chumash, published by Mesorah. This Chumash includes Rashi notes.

There are so many levels of Torah understanding. Those of us who learned the parshas in Hebrew school or Bible school learned by reading marvelous stories. As a child, I never got further than the events of the story. My adult understanding of Torah consists of the people and their characteristics, the situations and life lessons.

Women who have heard the Torah stories will enjoy this book for the parshas' deeper meaning and the connection to their lives. They will learn lessons of character trait improvement and develop increased understanding of self.

What is Yoga?
The word yoga means "union," referring to the mind, the body and the soul. Yoga is the practice of physical postures or poses that enhance stretching, balance, strength and flexibility.

Yoga is a routine for physical, mental, emotional and spiritual health. We discover ourselves on all these levels through our yoga practice. We physically do the exercises and make our bodies healthier by practicing on a regular basis. We pay attention and concentrate on our poses; our mind is focused on our yoga practice. We feel good about ourselves. We have accomplished our goals of a healthier body and enhanced concentration. A sound mind and a sound body augment our soul and encourage growth in positive directions. We develop our soul by becoming the best "me" that we can be using the tools of the mind and the body that were given to us. Yoga enhances the way we live with wisdom, insight, discernment, mindfulness and acceptance.

Why Together?

We are each created in God's image (Bereishis 9:26). All the attributes of God are one. We humans are one. Our mind, our body and our soul are encompassed in one entity. Our life goal is to be the best "one" that we can be using all of our qualities. We elevate the body to holiness by improving our character traits. We bring this wisdom to our physical selves. During life there is no separation of the body from the mind or the soul. We use the mind and the soul to sanctify the body. We need to protect and care for our body so that we can learn and develop to our highest abilities. The mind functions only in our body.

When the soul leaves the body, there is no further opportunity for growth of our minds or our spirit. This is the teaching of Torah. We are commanded to improve our character traits, or middos, by doing mitzvahs, or commandments. These mitzvahs are actions performed by our body. Doing mitzvahs is how we make our body holy. All human functions that engage the body and the mind are sanctified by mitzvahs. For example, we say a blessing over the food we eat, we make holy our life cycle events, and we watch our tongues so that we do not speak evil.

Yoga teaches mindfulness, concentration and oneness of mind, body and soul. Yoga postures improve our body, which allows our mind and soul to open and learn.

I have practiced yoga for more than twenty years and I have studied Torah for many years. The wisdoms of Torah and the benefits of yoga combine to enhance the learning of each. The concentration needed to do the yoga poses and the adaptability of each pose to the level of the student led me to a connection of yoga to the Torah. Just as we understand Torah at the level of learning we have reached, so we practice our yoga at the level of flexibility and strength of our body.

Many people learn physically. "They use touch, action and movement to learn. The same breathing and relaxation exercises of yoga helps them to focus and open their mind to new things. Focusing keeps people who are very physical calm, centered, relaxed and aware" (from the website learning-styles-online.com). This is known as kinesthetic learning or tactile learning. Learning takes place by carrying out a physical activity in addition to listening to a lecture or watching a demonstration. Perhaps you have had the experience where someone has shown you how to do something and you said, "Let me do it. I learn by doing it."

Focusing
Yoga teaches us to focus on what we are doing. Our mind is like a laser beam concentrating on the yoga position. Our aim is to maximize flexibility of our joints and increase the strength of our muscles. We try to be in the best posture for the pose and pay attention to our body parts so that the yoga practice is the most meaningful. Our mind is totally focused on the yoga movements and the yoga breath.

Focusing is a habit, just like many other characteristics. When we are in the habit of centering on our yoga practice, it spills over to other parts of our life. We will find that we are more in the moment and not daydreaming. We are attentive and aware. Our attention is in the present and not wandering.

"Monkey brain" is the brain that keeps a constant conversation going on in our head, even when we are doing something else. Sometimes, when we do our daily activities, study Torah, or when we say our prayers, the monkey brain keeps going. We speak the prayer, read the parsha, go to the store, but in our heads the monkey brain is going. "I have to make a shopping list, I have to clean the guest room, I need to make an appointment with the dentist, why did she say that and I should have said this." All of this is going on in our heads and it keeps on going regardless of what else we are doing. It takes away from the experience of what we are trying to do or to learn or to understand. Yoga will teach us how to stay focused and will keep the monkey brain at bay. We can have more meaningful prayers and Torah study. We can actively be in each moment of our day.

Parsha and Yoga focuses on using our God-given potential for growing and being our best: for taking ownership of our deeds, being responsible for our actions, and being considerate of others. Focusing our mind to have clarity of purpose, being mindful, fully conscious and aware of the present moment are lessons taken from yoga and applied to Torah study and daily prayer.

Our Purpose in Life
Our job in this world is to become the best "me" that we can be. We don't have to become the best person in the world, we just have to use what God gave us and use it well. There is a business expression that says "Don't leave anything on the table." This means that when you negotiate, don't give away what you don't have to give away. We are born with characteristics and abilities. What a crime to leave them unused "on the table."

Although God created the world and keeps creating everything that happens, we retain free will. We make the choices of how we will deal with the situations in our lives. We decide how they affect us.

Our yoga practice is the yoga practice that is best for our body. We each may do the same position but the way the position is done, the depth that the position is taken and the control in retaining the position is different. When we are doing yoga, we decide how far we can go in a position. We take our body to the maximum extension of the pose that we can do today. It may be different tomorrow when we may be a little more flexible or, perhaps, a little more tired. Our yoga practice is a daily accommodation to what is happening. Each of us makes our yoga practice unique, just as our lives are one of a kind.

Our trust in God is based on knowing that each of the events in our lives is for our benefit and that whatever happens is the best thing for us. It might not seem that way when it is happening and we might not always get the long view, but we know that our life is the life that we need to live. The lessons we are learning and the growth we are doing are the lessons and growth that are necessary for us to be our very best, to meet our potential.

My Torah knowledge comes from books and classes in Jewish studies. I am a ba'alas teshuva (a Jewish female from a secular background who becomes religiously observant in an Orthodox fashion later in life) and have practiced yoga for more than twenty years. The yoga practice that is best for beginners is one that emphasizes flexibility and stretching. Personally, I have downloaded several yoga audios to my computer and do my own yoga practice at home. Many videos and audios are available online and in shops. Find one you enjoy. If you find a class that is right for you, join it. Yoga works with repetition and should be practiced at least two times a week.

My goal is to make Torah interesting, relevant and accessible to more women. It is wonderful to teach Torah along with the physical and mental benefits of doing yoga. The word Torah means to teach and it is a mitzvah to learn Torah and to teach Torah (Deuteronomy 6:7). Join me in our study of yoga and the parsha of the week. Let me share with you my understanding and love of Torah and my appreciation for the benefits of yoga.

In *Parsha and Yoga* there is a sketch of the yoga pose and simple steps for the position. This book is not written to take the place of a yoga class. I strongly suggest that you find a class that you like and learn yoga with the personal attention you will receive from an instructor. The yoga pose that I selected for the parsha lesson will remind you of the message of the parsha of the week. Please consult your physician before you begin any exercise program.

Book I

Bereishis/Genesis

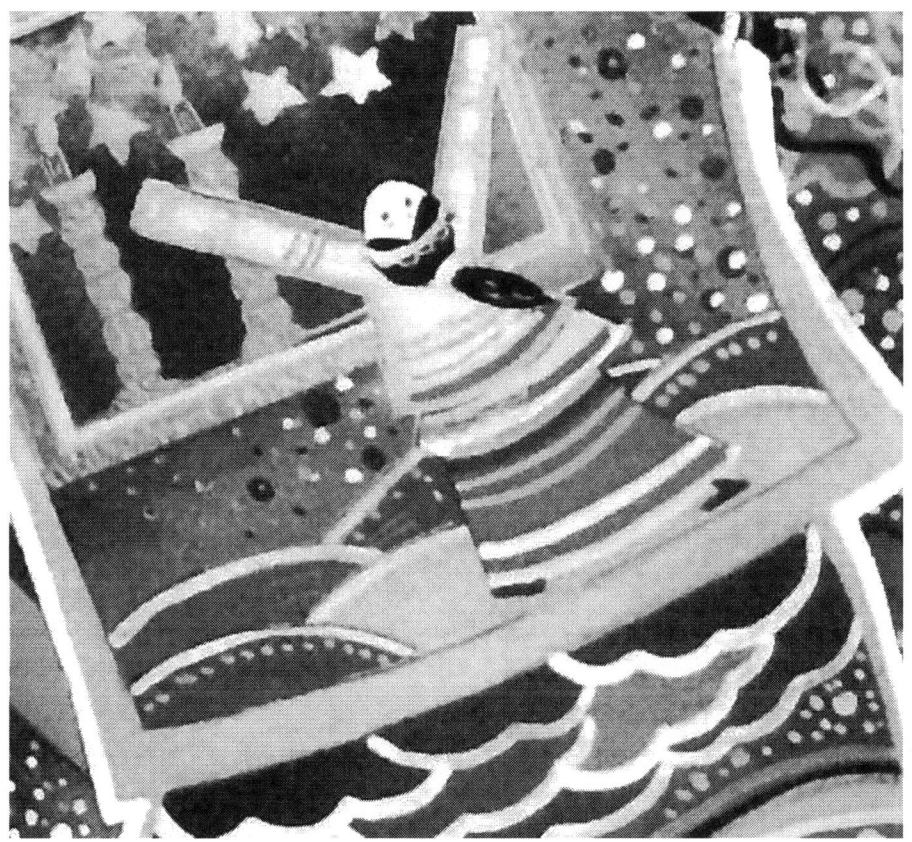

BEREISHIS (IN THE BEGINNING)

Parsha Insight — We have everything we need

"In the beginning God created the heaven and the earth."
The opening words of Torah are powerful. We are told, right from the start of Torah, that God created all and maintains all. We are here because of God's will.

"the earth was unformed and void, and darkness"
"and the spirit of God hovered"
In the beginning, there was nothing. Ramban, also known as Nachmanides (Rabbi Moshe ben Nachman, 13th century Spain), in the Chumash Ramban- Commentary on the Torah, in Genesis says, "...God created, from absolute nothingness, the prime matter of the earth and all that it would contain...in four forms: fire, water, earth and air." From this primary matter, all else was formed. Ramban also said that the specifics of the creation of the universe are not known to man. There are human limitations to accurately formulate or even imagine the presence of the origin of the universe (from *Awesome Creation* by Rabbi Yosef Bitton).

"And God said: 'Let there be light.' And there was light."
Where did this light come from? Not the sun, because it had not yet been created. The luminaries were not created until the fourth day. This is the light of the revelation of creation. And God saw the light, that it was good.

God Said and God Saw...
"God said..." refers to God created. The universe was created with Ten Utterances (*Pirkei Avos, Sayings of the Fathers*). "And God said: 'Let the waters beneath the heaven be gathered into one area, and let the dry land appear.'"

"God saw..." refers to God sustaining and continuing His involvement with His creation. "[A]nd God saw that it was good." This is not a one-time action. God is not backing off and letting us take over. At all times, God is keeping the energy and strength of the creation going.

On day six, Hashem created the animals. God said, "Let the earth bring forth living creatures...And God saw it was good."

When God created man, He did not say it was good. Instead God blessed man: "Be fruitful and multiply." Rambam, also known as Maimonides (Rabbi Moshe ben Maimon, Spain 12th century), says that this is because we are responsible for our actions. We have free will and needed a blessing so that we would make the proper choices.

"And God saw all that He had made, and behold it was very good." What made "all that He had made" very good? The individual creations were good, but the total, the combination of all, was very good. Everything fit; all the parts served each other. We could say that the interaction of the creations functioned together and was very good.

On the seventh day of creation, God rested. This is Shabbos, the most basic facet of Jewish life. "God blessed the seventh day and sanctified it because on it He abstained from all His work." My Shabbos is a day to regroup, reflect, connect with God, have a wonderful Shabbos meal and visit with friends. It is a time to be grateful for all my blessings. Shabbos is a gift. We are gifted with a day of no work.

Lessons of Bereishis
"Now the serpent was more subtle than any beast of the field."
Adam and Eve had everything they needed for a beautiful life in the Garden of Eden. "And God said: 'Behold, I have given you every herb yielding seed, which is upon the face of all the earth, and every tree, in which is the fruit of a tree yielding seed—to you it shall be for food; and to every beast of the earth, and to every fowl of the air, and to everything that creeps upon the earth...every green herb is for food.'"

Only one thing was unavailable to them. "...but of the tree of the knowledge of good and evil, you shall not eat of it; for in the day that you eat it you shall surely die."

Look at all our blessings. We have everything that we need. Most of us have more than we need, and the urge to get more is our undoing. Are we being led by our desires for more? Is the yetzer hora (the snake, the evil inclination) encouraging us to get another car, a bigger house, more clothing? Adam and Eve lost the bountiful Garden of Eden, were forced to work for their bread, and came to know death. While touching the Tree of Knowledge or eating its fruit did not lead to immediate death it did take away their immortality.

"And the man said: 'The woman whom you gave me, she gave me of the tree, and I did eat.'
"And the woman said: 'The serpent beguiled me, and I did eat.'"
When Adam was confronted by God he said that the woman you gave me made me do it. He put the blame on Eve and did not take responsibility for his own actions. Rashi says that this is Adam's lack of gratitude to God for giving him Eve. We learn in Torah to take ownership of our acts. Everything we do has repercussions and it is not someone else's fault that we pursued a negative path.

Adam and Eve were seduced by their wants. The snake represents the wants and desires of man. The snake symbolizes the seduction of greed, the arrogance of ego and the hatefulness of jealousy. As we go through Torah, we will see that these three negative characteristics are continuously causing people trouble. When greed, arrogance and jealousy take over, we are making free-will choices of negative behavior. This is compounded by justifying our actions and saying it was someone else's fault.

"And the Lord had respect unto Abel and to his offering; but unto Cain and to his offering He had not respect." Cain brought flax as an offering to God and Abel brought the firstborn from his flock. Cain's offering was rejected not because it was inferior in quality. It was rejected because of the spirit behind the offering. Cain had free choice and took the wrong path. He was responsible for his actions and had it in his power to improve himself. Instead, Cain got even more angry and jealous and killed his brother. Cain killing Abel shows us the evil consequences of jealousy. When one is jealous, he loses his mind and is capable of horrendous acts.

If you are interested in more about creation, I recommend *Genesis and the Big Bang* (Bantam 1990) by Gerald Lawrence Schroeder, an Orthodox Jewish physicist, author, lecturer and teacher. Another recommendation is *Awesome Creation* (Gefen Publishing House 2013) by Rabbi Yosef Bitton.

Yoga—Basic seated pose

You have everything you need to practice yoga.
Take responsibility for your yoga practice and make it "yours" by adapting the poses to suit your body.
Be grateful for all that you have.
Make the freewill decision to be the best you that you can be.

Sit on the yoga mat.
You may want to sit on the edge of a folded blanket.
Cross your legs, like you did in camp as a kid.
Try to get your knees close to the ground.
Do not force or strain.
Our hands are on our knees with palms up.
We are receptive to our yoga practice just as we are receptive to Torah learning.
Eyes closed and breathe deeply through the nose.
Re-cross your legs with the other leg closer to your body.
Relax, close your eyes, inhale and exhale through the nose.
This pose is good for stress reduction.
It is a calming pose. The pose helps us develop patience.

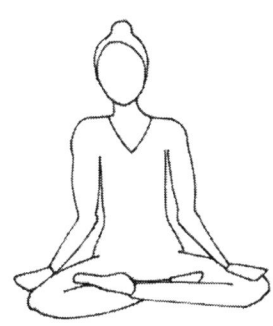

Noah (rest or comfort)

Parsha Insight–Use your potential

"Noah was a righteous man, perfect for his generations."
Noah lived in a generation of people without moral fiber. He followed the basic laws of moral, human behavior. (These are called the Noahide Laws, basic societal laws for all the world.) Noah, compared to all the other people, was a righteous man.

The seven Noahide Laws.
Do not worship idols.
Do not curse God.
Do not murder.
Do not commit adultery or incest.
Do not steal.
Establish courts of justice.
Do not eat the flesh of a living animal.

The Noahide Laws are not accepted like Torah, they are part of being human. Imagine the level of depravity if the people were violating the Noahide Laws. Ten generations have passed since the creation of Adam, whose descendants tainted the world with immorality, idolatry and stealing. Things were so bad that God could see no alternative to wiping out everything with a flood that destroyed all of earth's life. Only Noah, his family and the animals needed to repopulate the earth would remain.

When God told him that there would be a flood and all would perish, and to build an Ark for himself, his family and the designated animals, Noah followed all of God's explicit instructions. It took Noah a long time to build the Ark and people came by and asked him what he was doing. He said he was building an Ark because there was going to be a flood.

He did not encourage others to better behavior or implore them to change their ways. Noah knew better, but he was silent. He did nothing extra. He certainly did not live up to his potential. He did no teaching about moral behavior or about God. He did not beg God for mercy, to save the lives of the people. He remained silent. Even though the people were immoral, it seems drastic to destroy everything and just save Noah.

Did Noah think there would be no room on the Ark for anybody else? Did he, maybe, not believe that God would actually bring the flood? Perhaps Noah thought the Ark was his reward for his morality. Perhaps this was the way that God was providing to save him and his family and the animals to continue life on earth. Maybe the Ark was a way to keep Noah and his family separate from the rest of humanity and their immorality. Noah doesn't seem to care much for anyone other than his family.

Noah's halfhearted warning that a flood was coming did not have much conviction to it. It did not seem as though Noah was fully committed because he did not even enter the Ark until he was forced to by the height of the waters. These actions do not show an unshakable belief in the coming flood. Noah would follow God's instructions and build the Ark, but he wasn't ready to get in it without more proof. He needed to get really wet before he was convinced.

Do we do just enough so that there are no complaints? Do we pride ourselves that, compared to the rest of the population, we are pretty good? We need to live up to God's declaration after creation: the world was very good. Strive for "very good." Good enough is the bare minimum. When we are very good we are achieving a high degree of performance, we are extremely proficient, we are exceeding the levels we thought possible. We realize the potential that God has given us.

When the waters began to recede Noah sent out a dove to see if there was dry land. The dove returned with an olive leaf in its mouth. This is a figurative representation connecting the physical world and the spiritual. It is symbolic because the oil of an olive tree is used for light and light means wisdom. God destroyed the world with a flood because of the evil of the people. Noah and his family now have an opportunity to start anew with the wisdom from before the flood. Upon leaving the Ark, Noah got a blessing, "Be fruitful and multiply and fill the land." This is the same blessing that Adam got, to people the land. God made a covenant with Noah to rebuild humanity.

Noah shamed himself, got drunk and exhibited indecent behavior. He did not live up to his potential. Success is scary, and many people get to the brink of achieving it and then mess up. Noah worked so hard to keep the animals alive and to keep his family together. He was blessed by God and received a covenant of the eternal rainbow (the sign of the rainbow is God's promise that He will never again destroy the earth by water for man's sins). What did he do? He messed up, got drunk and shamed himself.

Noah saw the errors of his ways and prophesied that the generations from his son, Shem, would be the Children of Israel. It took ten generations from Noah to Abraham. Many comparisons are made between the two men. Noah could have been our Abraham if he had only taken the opportunity to teach people how to mend their ways and to share with them his understandings of God. Noah followed the instructions of God but went no further. He did not leave the comfort of his own family or extend himself to others. The name Noah means rest or comfort. Abraham taught people about monotheism and showed them the value of moral behavior. Noah missed his chance of really being great.

Terry in "On the Waterfront" says, "You don't understand. I coulda had class. I coulda been a contender. I coulda been a somebody..." What a great catastrophe when one discovers that not "being a somebody" is due to laziness, bad habits or negative influences in life. Our job is to take our traits and our skills and use them to our fullest ability. That's employing our God-given potential to become the best person that we can be.

How can we improve? Look at the gifts we are born with: our intelligence, our bodily abilities, our talents and our personality traits. Are they being utilized fully? Are we really smart, but we take the easy way out and read popular novels, not challenging our brain with heavier reading? Are we physically strong and healthy and eat junk food and too much of it, allowing ourselves to get out of shape and to develop digestive problems? Are we not so generous, and find excuses for why we can't give more charity? We can change.

Make goals that are realistic and achievable. Be sure that each goal is flexible, with a little wiggle room, so that we can accommodate to the events that will happen. And things will happen. Set up goals in small steps so that we can mark off points of achievement. Nothing is more rewarding than checks on our list.

Sometimes we are on the wrong path and our plans don't work. It's okay to go back, revisiting a preceding step and make changes. That's what being flexible is about. We don't give up because one step is not possible, we look around and find something else. Depend on intuition to see if we are working towards a proper goal for ourselves. When we utilize our potential we are achieving our vision. Things take time. Don't rush or force events. We trust in God and do our hishtadlus (we do our part). Accept where we are right now and enjoy the process. What a marvelous goal: to be the best me that I can be!

Parsha and Yoga

Yoga–Cobbler position

The cobbler puts together, makes and fixes shoes following the designer's plans and instructions.
Noah followed God's instructions and made the Ark.
The cobbler yoga position is restful and comfortable.

Sit on your mat, legs out.
You may want to sit on the edge of a folded blanket.
Bring your feet towards your pelvis.
Soles of the feet together.
Knees down but do not force.
Hold your feet with your hands.
To release, stretch out legs, one at a time.
Great for relaxing stomach.

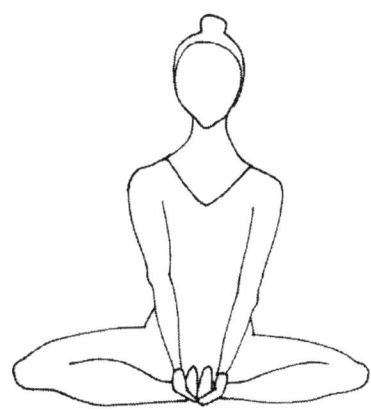

Lech Lecha (go for yourself)

Parsha Insight—Go towards something

We now come to a pivotal point in our history. Twenty generations have passed from Adam to Abraham, including the ten generations from Noah to Abraham. Abraham was born in the year 1948 from creation. The spiritual level of man is again in decline. These first two thousand years from creation are known as the Age of Desolation (torah.org Parsha Perceptions by Rabbi Pinchas Winston).

Abraham, coming from an idol-making family, looked at life around him and understood that there can only be one God. The idols that man made from wood or stone could not be gods. The sun and the moon had to get their attributes from someplace. All had to come about from one God.

Monotheism was not a new idea in Abraham's time. People knew about God and considered idols as a means of transmission to God. Idols were used as an intermediary to God and were thought to have powers of their own. Abraham's mission was to teach people that God is One and that no intermediaries are necessary. Abraham is also known for his kindness and is considered the grandfather of all Jews.

God told Abraham to "Go for yourself from your land, from your relatives and from your father's house to the land that I will show you." The order of leaving cuts ties gradually. First Abraham leaves his country or homeland, then his family and friends, and finally his father and intimate connections.

When we make big changes in our lives, it helps if we can make a gradual adjustment. Major life events, unfortunately, are not gradual. They come about from crisis, trauma, catastrophe or the turning points of life such as marriage, the birth of a child or the death of a loved one. In a life-defining moment, everything seems to change.

In this parsha we are given the good advice to make changes gradually and to try, if possible, not to overhaul our lives all at once. Slow the process down and try to make it transitional rather than abrupt. Take time to accommodate the changes and allow yourself to grow from the situation.

Abraham is told to "Go for yourself," to go for his own benefit. Abraham obeyed without question, showing his devotion and trust. Abraham went with Sarah and "the souls they made" (their disciples) to the land that God showed them, which was Canaan or Israel. Going for yourself is for your own benefit. It is not running away from; it is going towards. God will make Abraham a "great nation," but this could not happen in Haran (his father's home).

After twenty-seven years working for a major insurance company, I realized that a change was necessary for my personal growth. I needed the challenge of self-employment. I left my corporate job and opened a retail bead store. This enabled me to develop different skills and to use abilities that were dormant as an employee in a large corporation. I got closer to my essential self. This was a period of tremendous growth for me.

Beading and jewelry-making had been my hobby, and being able to turn it into a business was a dream come true. I did not think I was unique and believed that many other people would love to take a hobby, something they do for enjoyment, and turn it into a way to earn a living. I taught "How to Take Your Hobby and Turn It into a Business" at adult education classes. One point I stressed: do not leave your current position because you are running away from a bad situation. Leave because you are going to something better with more opportunities. This is going for yourself.

Magen Avraham (Shield of Abraham)
These words form the end of the first blessing of Shemoneh Esrei, the Amidah or standing prayer. God says, "I will make you into a great nation, I will bless you, and I will exalt your name; and you will be a blessing." You will have children and grandchildren, the generations coming from them, and they will form a nation. You will be blessed and exalted, and you will forever be seen as a blessing. Magen Avraham. This is God's blessing and promise to Abraham. Adam and Noah were blessed by God. Abraham was blessed and also told that he will be a blessing to others. God will curse those who curse Abraham and bless those who bless Abraham. God also gave Abraham the power to bless others.

In words that foreshadow the Jews leaving Egypt with Moses, God says, "I am the God who took you out of Ur." In this parsha God repeats many times the promise of the land of Israel and the making of Abraham a "great nation":

12:2   "And I will make of you a great nation"
12:7   "To your offspring I will give this land"
13:15   "For all the land that you see"
13:16   your offspring will be as numerous as the dust of the earth (I'm paraphrasing)
15:5   your offspring will be as numerous as the stars (I'm paraphrasing)
15:7   "To give you this land to inherit it"
15:18   "To your descendants have I given this land"
17:7   "I will give to you and to your offspring after you the land…the whole of the land of Canaan"

Abraham asked God how he would know that this was the land for the Children of Israel. Was Abraham doubting God? Maybe the Children of Israel would not deserve the land? Was this promise of the land dependent upon the acts of himself and his offspring? What if they sinned?

God responds that Abraham's children would be strangers in a land not their own and, referring to the Egyptian exile, that they will be enslaved. "Know with certainty that your offspring shall be aliens in a land not their own—and they will serve them, and they will oppress them—four hundred years. But also the nation that they will serve, I shall judge, and afterwards they will leave with great wealth."

When you read "he sojourned—he stayed," not "he lived," it means just passing through on the way to the land that God promised Abraham.

Yoga–Easy seated waist turn

Abraham turned his disciples towards the Oneness of God.

Easy seated waist turn
Start A: Sit sideways in a chair on the right side.
Inhale.
Turn right, exhale, hands to chair back.
Inhale, turn back to start A.
Start B: Sit sideways in a chair on the left side.
Inhale.
Now, turn left, exhale, hands to chair back.
Inhale, turn back to start B.
Great easy stretching pose.

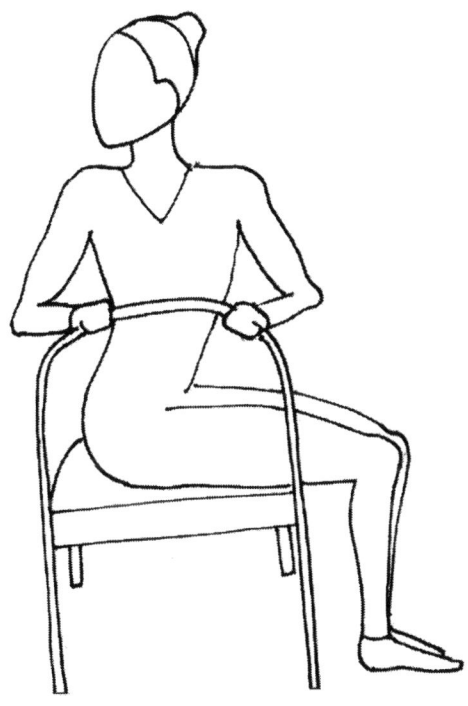

Vayeira (and he appeared)

Parsha Insight — Run to do kindness

Mitzvah to Visit the Sick
Hashem came to visit Abraham on the third day after his circumcision. Recovery from bris milah is the most painful on day three.

Run to Do Kindness
Abraham was sitting at the tent entrance looking for guests so that he could do a kindness. When Abraham saw that three guests were arriving, he ran to greet them. Even though he was recovering from surgery, he still was on the lookout for occasions to do a mitzvah. Abraham did not delay in doing a mitzvah, he "ran" to do an act of kindness. Not only are we to look for opportunities to do a kindness, we are to do the mitzvah promptly and with happiness.

Abraham, himself, arranged for the food and drink for the guests and was very giving in his acts of kindness to the strangers. He asked a servant to bring some water so that the three men could wash their feet. Abraham was not as accommodating with the water as he was with the food and drink.

He believed that the guests were idol worshipers and he knew that idol worshipers worshiped the dust on their feet. Abraham did not want this dust on his property. From this we learn to be slightly wary of strangers and to find out more before we are completely open with them. Washing the feet was not an act of honor. It was a precaution.

These acts are precursors of future events. What Abraham himself did for his guests, Hashem (God) did for the Jews in the desert. Abraham was the one who made sure that the guests had food. Hashem directly fed the people with manna (food from heaven). Abraham had a servant bring the water for the guests' feet. Hashem had the rock bring water. Like Abraham, Hashem delegated the bringing of the water.

Is this suggesting that Abraham should not have been somewhat suspicious of the strangers? Perhaps this is to remind us that everything is not always readily available and water, in the desert, is certainly scarce. We should not be completely generous to our own detriment. Have a good eye, see people in a good light; still be aware that you don't know the whole story. If you have a suspicion, like Abraham who thought the men were idol worshipers and wanted the dust from their feet removed before they rested on his property, go slowly, take precautions and reserve judgment. As with most middos, find the proper balance in your behavior.

God Talks to Himself
"And Hashem said, 'Shall I conceal from Abraham what I do...' Seemingly, God is talking to himself and resolving to tell Abraham He loves him, and that his offspring and dependents would survive the evil in the world. Abraham merits this because he taught his children and commanded his household regarding charity and justice. Children are taught not only by words but most importantly by example. Abraham's mission in the world was told in Lech Lecha. Abraham will be made a great nation and he will be blessed.

Lot a Weak Man
Lot, a relative of Abraham, was not an evil man but he was a weak man. When he arrived in Sodom, he sat at the gates. In those times, only the great men sat at the gates. Remember the Purim story and that Mordecai sat at the gates. Lot was weak and as time went on, he moved from the gates of Sodom to the city, and from the city until he was in the midst of everything that was happening. Lot did not realize his own vulnerability to evil.

This is something we all have to be aware of. If you live and deal with evil people, it is almost as if the evil is catching. We all have heard the expression, "Birds of a feather flock together." We are all vulnerable to our environment and we must choose our friends and associates with care.

Din and Nissayon
When God dealt with Sodom it was through din. Din is judgment. Sodom was an evil place and the people were evil. We understand the cause and effect of the judgment and the reasons that the city and its people were destroyed.

When God told Abraham to bring his son, Isaac, as an offering, it is nissayon. A nissayon makes no sense to us. It is beyond our understanding. Abraham understood that this was God's test and that any argument would have been for naught. We are not Abraham and are bewildered by God's request.

What exactly was God testing? Was it to see if Abraham would obey God without question? Was God looking for a stronger belief than just performing a task unquestioned? Remember, Noah performed his tasks. Noah did what God asked him to do.

Hashem asked Abraham to bring his son, his only one, whom he loves, Isaac, as an offering. In parshas Lech Lecha, Hashem makes a Covenant of Parts with Abraham and tells him that he will be a great nation; that he will have children and grandchildren coming from them; that they will be as numerous as the stars. Many times Hashem tells Abraham that he is blessed and that a nation will come from his generations. Abraham had asked how he would know that the Promised Land (Israel) would be given to the Jewish people. Hashem needed to see if Abraham had the emuna and the trust in God that was necessary to know that from his generations would come the nation of Jews.

Abraham was told to bring Isaac as an offering for the final test of Abraham's emuna. Hashem did not say sacrifice; He said "offering." Offering is the act of presentation while sacrifice is the act of forgoing. Abraham understood the test and did not argue with Hashem. Abraham did have the emuna and trusted that the generations of the Jewish Nation would come from him.

The Trial of the Akeida
The Akeida—the binding of Isaac—is Abraham's trial. Seems as though Isaac had a lot invested. Why aren't we calling it Isaac's trial? After the Akeida and the appearance of the sacrificial ram, Isaac goes on with his life. What happens to Abraham?

Before the Akeida, Abraham was preoccupied with the external world, with his disciples and his negotiations with world powers. After the Akeida, Abraham is more involved with family. Rambam says that he concentrates on his mission to his family and the building of the Jewish Nation through Isaac.

Yoga—Deeper seated twist

Let's sit at the door of our tent, turning right and left, looking for guests and acts of kindness that we can do.
This pose is more advanced than the easy seated waist turn in parshas Lech Lecha.

Sit on the mat with your legs out.
You may want to sit on the edge of a folded blanket.
Bend the right knee.
Right foot flat on ground.
Right hand on the ground behind you.
Left arm to the outside of the right knee.
Twist right.
Hold for at least two breaths.
Return to center.
Change sides.
As you grow in your yoga practice, you may be able to hold a position for five breaths.

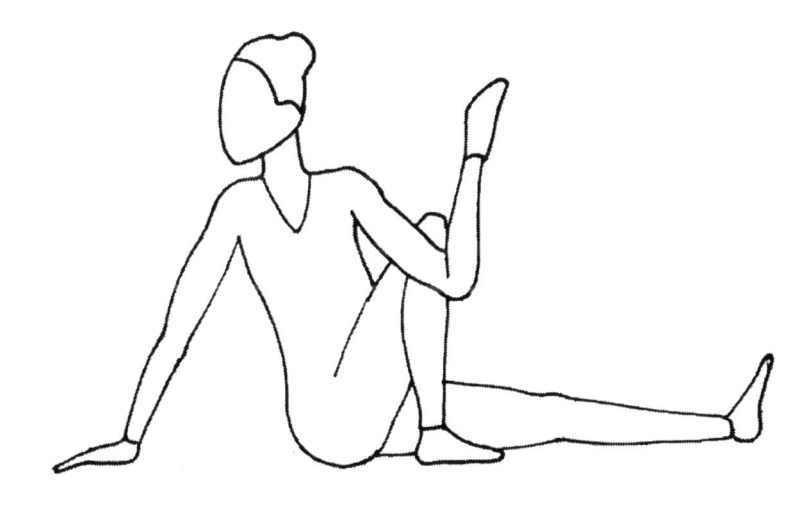

Chayei Sarah (life of Sarah)

Parsha Insight—Every minute counts

The parsha opens with the line, "Sarah's lifetime was one hundred years, twenty years, and seven years; the years of Sarah's life." This is a very unusual way to tell us that Sarah died at the age of one hundred and twenty-seven years. The repetition of the word years is to tell us that every year, every minute of Sarah's life was important. She did not waste or spend foolishly the precious time of her holy life. In Rashi's words, "all of them (the years) were equal in their goodness." Sarah lived a sin-free and perfect life and in her merit, Queen Esther (from the Purim story), her descendant, presided over one hundred and twenty-seven provinces.

Later on in our parsha study we will come to Jacob and how he saw his life and his time in this world. These stories remind us that it is up to us to appreciate time and to use it wisely. Every moment of our lives is precious and not to be wasted. Time, once spent, cannot be regained. Think of the things someone could do if two, three hours a day were not spent watching television.

This point is illustrated by this story from the Jewish Press, "Time is Precious" by Menachem Ben-Mordechai (May 31, 2013): "Once, the Chofetz Chaim was waiting with a student for a train. He said to the talmid [student], 'Please take a sefer [book] out of the bag and we will learn together.' The talmid checked the time and saw the train was scheduled to arrive very soon. He said, 'Rebbe, the train's coming in five minutes'—meaning that it's a bit of a tircha (burden) to get the sefer for such a short amount of time. The Chofetz Chaim responded, 'It is true that the train is coming in five minutes, but there are also five minutes until the train comes.'"

Why Did Sarah Die?
Since the story of Sarah's death is right after the Akeida (the binding of Isaac), they must be connected. The Torah does not tell us the events immediately preceding Sarah's death, but there are four midrashic narratives (stories by rabbinic sages) that we can review.

Midrash is a form of storytelling that explores ethics and values. It takes a posik (verse) from Torah and interprets the sentence to explain what happened. The following midrashic stories are possible events that may have occurred prior to Sarah's death. Each of the stories has a particular outlook based upon the ethical value it is trying to convey.
Sarah was told by Satan that Abraham slaughtered Isaac. This caused her so much grief that she died. The question is raised, in Sarah's mind, of whether it was possible that Abraham would sacrifice Isaac and that Hashem would not intervene.

Sarah heard about the Akeida and also that Isaac did not die. She did not know that a ram was sent by Hashem to spare Isaac. She was devastated to think that Isaac disobeyed his father and was overwhelmed by grief that Isaac was not loyal to God.

Her time was up. She lived a full and holy life for one hundred and twenty seven years. Sarah died proud of Abraham's trust in Hashem and proud of Isaac's willingness to obey his father. Sarah had accomplished her mission on earth and was ready to die.

When Abraham was tested by Hashem he was told gradually and gently so that he had time to get used to the test: "Please, take your son, your only one, whom you love, Isaac...and bring him up there as an offering..." This was Abraham's test and he had the resolve to obey. It was not Sarah's test and she had no storehouse of fortitude. Sarah was not told gradually and did not have the opportunity to prepare herself. Sarah was told bluntly, and perhaps incompletely, about the Akeida and was overcome by grief.

Many things are better when accepted in small doses rather than all at once. If you are learning Torah and taking on mitzvahs, do it gradually, like climbing steps. At each new level, pause and make the new mitzvah(s) part of your life. Then continue moving forward.

Yoga—Downward dog in small steps

If you are not familiar with the yoga poses, it is best to begin very gently and gradually become more accomplished in each pose. A gradual introduction to downward dog is kind to your body.

Start by bending from the hips.
This is a ninety degree or right angle bend.
It is not a downward dog bend.
This is a partial downward bend.
It is okay to have your knees bent.

If you are not dizzy with this partial inversion, progress to tabletop.
You are on your hands and knees.
Head in straight line with spine.

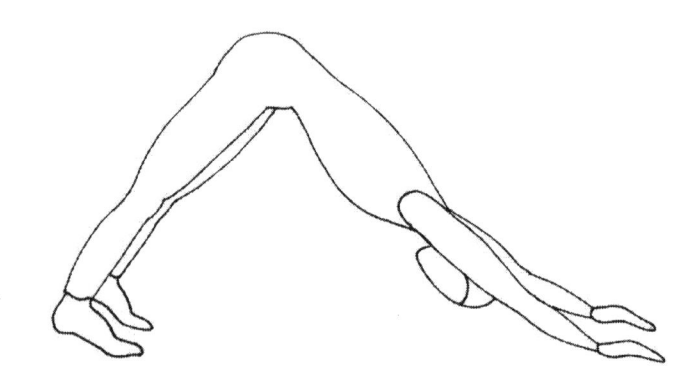

When you are ready, push back, weight on hands.
Hips up, head down, like a V inverted.
Your feet are pressing down, they do not have to be flat on the ground.
Your knees could be bent.

As you progress:
Your hips push back more.
Your back is straighter.
Your head hangs between your shoulders.
Your heels are lowering to the ground.
Your legs are straighter.

Toldos (generations)

Parsha Insight—Heredity or environment

Hashem Heard His Prayers
Both Rivka and Isaac prayed for children. Hashem heard Isaac's prayers. What happened to Rivka's prayers?

Isaac's prayers were heard by God because of his yichas, which is his inherited factors and his genealogical family line. The prayers of a righteous person, born from a righteous person, are greater than the prayers of a righteous person born from a family of sinful people. When praying for personal benefit, the scales are in the favor of the one with yichas. The merits of the one praying and those who came before him are combined with respect to prayers for individual favor.

Both Isaac and Rivka were righteous people. Rivka came from a sinful family and had to work hard to overcome her background. Shouldn't that count extra? When praying on behalf of the community or all the Jewish people, the merit of the one who rose over and above his line of birth is counted greater than the prayers of the person with yichas.

Hashem had made a covenant with Abraham. "You will have children and grandchildren, the generations coming from them, and they will form a nation." Isaac and Rivka would have children at the right time. Three of the four Matriarchs—Sarah, Rivka and Rachel—had trouble conceiving. It is said that this was because God wanted their prayers, and they all prayed for many years for children. Each matriarch eventually conceived.

Isaac is Gevurah

Isaac is identified with gevurah, which is power, strength and discipline. Fighting and resisting so that we can have our own way is weakness. It is an appeal to our physical and egotistical needs. Isaac's strength is evident in his negotiations with the Philistines. He knows when to speak and when to be quiet. He knows that making arrangements with someone who does not even comprehend the meaning of peace, the topic of negotiation, is futile.

Isaac was not only graced with good yichas, he was a tzaddik (great Torah person) in his own right. Isaac is known for his awe of Hashem. He is one of the Avos (patriarchs). In Shemoneh Esrei we say "God of Abraham, God of Isaac and God of Jacob." Abraham is known for kindness, Isaac for strength, and Jacob for truth.

Rivka Perfected Her Middos

Rivka could not change her family background. She could and did perfect her middos, her character traits. In the Torah, we first meet Rivka at the well, where her consideration for Eliezer and his camels is immediately seen. Eliezer knows she would be a perfect wife for Isaac.

We can change and grow; we can overcome our family background. We can learn more in Torah and improve our middos. The key is to stay away from evil companions. Find people with the characteristics you want to emulate and make them your associates.

Twins But Different

Rivka had twins, Esau and Jacob. Both children were born to Isaac and Rivka. Both sons from the same gene pool. Both grew up in the same household. The difference in their nature was evident even in the womb. The parsha tells us that Rivka felt lots of movement during her pregnancy. Hashem told Rivka, "Two nations are in your womb..." One son, Esau, was wild and earthy and the other son, Jacob, was quiet and studious.

Esau and Jacob are like Isaac and the Philistines. "Two Nations" that don't even accept the same definition of the word peace. Each son had his own identity but they operated in different spheres. Esau is body and physical drives. Jacob is mind and soul. Twins, because one without the other is not complete. The twins are repeated in each of us. This is the striving to balance our physical side with our spiritual side.

Heredity or Environment
What is more important in the development of an individual, his genes or his environment? The birth and development of Esau and Jacob does not answer this question. Rather we see the repetition of the theme of the physically based son verses the spiritually based son. We have Cain and Abel, Ishmael and Isaac, and Esau and Jacob. One son is fit to have his offspring build the Jewish Nation and one is not.

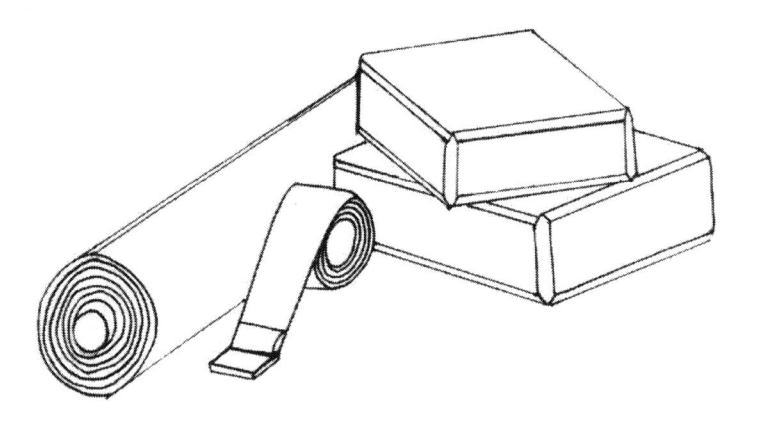

Yoga—Your yoga workout is yours

Just as each of our personalities differ because of heredity and environment, each of our bodies is different. Our body structure makes some yoga positions more natural and easier. It is important that you adapt the yoga pose to your figure. Become more in tune with your body and the way it moves. Your shape may cause you some limitations in the poses and the depth of the poses. No problem. Just alter the pose so that it is more comfortable for your body. Your yoga workout is "yours" and you should make changes to the position so that it is comfortable for your body.

Maybe a position is not comfortable at first. You can see that with practice, you will get to a point that the pose is easier. This is not the same as painful. If the position is painful, do not do it. The difference between pain and soreness is intensity. If you feel sore, it is a dull and uncomfortable feeling in the muscles. Pain is sharp and can be felt in the joints and muscles. Pain in not normal and you should stop your yoga practice. See your doctor if the pain persists.

Look into some yoga props to help you in the poses. A block and a strap are used by many to enhance the practice. See what the prop does for you and then decide if it is helpful. Try the strap to hold your leg up or to the side. The block is good for the triangle pose; it brings the ground a little closer. Be your own yoga guide and see what works for you.

Vayeitzei (and he went out)

Parsha Insight—Proper balance faith and personal effort

Evening Prayer
Jacob left his parents' home. On the way he "encountered the place" where Abraham bound Isaac. It was sundown and he prayed. Jacob established evening prayer, Maariv, which is a more informal prayer than the morning or afternoon prayers. The evening prayer is short, maybe taking ten or fifteen minutes. The night is approaching and it is a good time to reflect on the events that occurred that day.

Behold
Jacob slept. "And behold!" Hashem was there and told him that the ground which he was lying on would belong to his descendants. He was told his offspring would be as the dust of the earth and they would spread out in all directions. God said, "Behold, I am with you." Jacob knew, even though he was traveling with no riches, his help would come from Hashem and he had nothing to fear because God promised to guard him wherever he would go.

God assured Jacob that He will return him to the soil of Israel. Jacob knew his faith and his trust had to be balanced with his hishtadlus (personal effort). We see this in the many years he worked for Lavan. Jacob knew that God was with him regardless of Lavan's deceit and evil acts. Lavan made agreements and changed them; made promises and ignored them, and was definitely not a person to be trusted. God protected Jacob and gave him the tools to deal with Lavan.

Proper Balance
It is often a major trial for each of us to find proper balance. This has been my greatest personal challenge. I have always been a proactive type of person. It just seems natural to push forward and make something happen.

Over the years, I have learned to have more patience. I have seen how God weaves the events of my life together for the best results. Working hard and taking action is a necessary thing; Hashem wants our efforts. But there is a point where we need to pause and know that our lives depend on Hashem more than anything else.

How did I learn this? By watching things happen and trusting in Hashem. If God was leading me in a particular direction, if things began to fall into place, I knew I was on the right path. In the vernacular we say, "Go with the flow."

Lavan's Greeting
Lavan ran to Jacob and hugged and kissed him. He was "patting him down" to see what he had on him since Jacob appeared to arrive empty-handed. Being greeted is nice. Being patted down is not. We need to recognize the good in the bad and the bad in the good and understand its purpose.

Who is this person? What do they want from me? What is the situation that we are meeting? What happened before we met? What is the reputation of these people? Why am I here? What do I want? Loads of questions. We have trust in God that all that occurs is best for us.

At the same time, it is our responsibility to apply effort to discern the events and their impact on our lives. Our effort is to get as much information as we can so that we can evaluate properly. Our free will is the impact we allow events to have on our lives.

Jacob's Lesson
This is what Jacob learned: We must protect ourselves from evil people. Having a "good eye" for an evil person is not wise and not a virtue. Torah tells us to protect ourselves from evil people.

Lavan tells Jacob, "It is not done in our place to give the younger one (in marriage) before the older." This is sarcasm and should be a red flag that the speaker has evil intent. Lavan was giving an excuse for his deceit and deriding Jacob as the younger one who took Esau's blessings.

Jacob's Leaving
After many years of working for Lavan and dealing with his deceitful ways, Jacob left. Lavan pursued Jacob, caught up with him, and threatened Jacob. First, he said that Jacob should not have sneaked away. He should have allowed Lavan to throw a goodbye party.

Then he said that he could do evil to him and exert power over him. Anyone who threatens you, verbally or physically, is trying to control you and defeat you. This person is not thinking about you and is only applying pressure to overpower you.

God came to Lavan and told him, "Beware that you do not speak to Jacob either good or bad." According to Rashi, God is telling Lavan to stay away because good from a bad person is still bad. Torah is telling us that anything from an evil source is suspect. A wise person needs to be cautious and discerning. In the fourth blessing of the weekday Shemoneh Esrei prayer we ask for wisdom, insight and discernment. Our job, our hishtadlus, is to use our wisdom to protect ourselves and stay away from evil.

At the end of the parsha, "Lavan went and returned to his place. Jacob went on his way." They formed a truce, a pact, and went their own ways.

Yoga—Resting pose for pause and peace

Restorative or resting pose is a position of slowing down, pausing and peace. It is a fitting position for this parsha because Jacob established evening prayer. Both resting pose and prayer are very good before bedtime.

In addition to the established prayers, try hisbodedus, private personal prayers. Using your own words, pray to God. Tell Him about your day and about why you did or said things. Be honest. It is just you and God, and He already knows the truth. Ask for wisdom and the ability to discern truth. Be grateful for all you have and thank God. This is for you.

Say your thoughts. Whisper them and give your thoughts form. You will surprise yourself by the difference between thinking and whispering. Thinking is air; saying is concrete.

The resting pose is usually the last pose in a yoga practice. Time to rest and be grateful. Consider your blessings.

Lie on your back, flat on your mat, feet flop outward.
Hands at your side, palms up.
Long, slow and full inhales and exhales.
Relax.
Get up from the ground properly.
Roll gently to your right side.
Place both hands on the ground.
Push yourself up to a seated position.

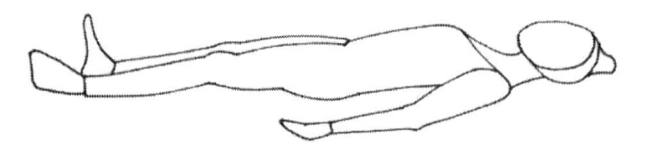

Vayishlach (and he sent)

Parsha Insight — Dealing with an adversary

Sending a Message
After thirty-four years away, Jacob returned home. He sent angels ahead of him with a message to Esau. In his message Jacob said that he had sojourned with Lavan.

The message to Esau conveyed two things. First, by living with Lavan, Jacob learned how to deal with an evil person. He learned how to protect himself from deceit. In parsha Vayeitzei Jacob protected himself in his work arrangement with Lavan. He made sure that odd-colored animals were born and, in accordance with their agreement, those he kept. Jacob learned the art of negotiation and the cunning needed to deal with a deceitful person.

The second part of the message is that throughout the twenty years with Lavan, Jacob kept the ways of his father and grandfather. He remained a righteous man.

Esau Has Four Hundred Men
The angels report that Esau was quickly heading towards Jacob with an army of four hundred men.

Dealing with an Adversary
Jacob's method of dealing with his brother has become a textbook model for how Jews have dealt with adversaries throughout history using prayer, appeasement, and battle.

Speak politely and show respect.
Jacob prepared for the meeting with Esau by wording the message to show respect. "To my lord, to Esau, so said your servant, Jacob."
Jacob was polite and respectful in the message and upon meeting Esau.

Bribe the other party with gifts.
Let them know why it is to their benefit not to instigate war.
Jacob gave Esau gifts. "I have oxen and donkeys, I am sending them to my lord..."

Pray to Hashem.
Know that the outcome is in the hands of Hashem.

Show strength.
Do your hishtadlus.
Jacob separated his convoy so that it appeared huge and as if he would be strong enough to overcome any force of Esau's.

Plenty vs. Everything

When Jacob and Esau met, Esau said he had plenty and Jacob said he had everything. The person who sees the purpose of life as physically acquiring things weighs his worth by what he has. He measures it and assesses it to establish his value. Having plenty means that on a scale of zero to a trillion, "I got plenty."

The person who is more involved with spiritual growth and personal development sees material things merely as what is needed for life. His value is his middos and not his money. Having everything is, "Whatever I need to live decently, I have."

Jacob Wary of Esau

Jacob prayed to Hashem to help him regardless of the outcome. Jacob saw two dangers in warring with Esau. The first was the possibility of actual war and the death of himself and his children. This would destroy the offspring whom Hashem promised would build the Jewish Nation. Even though Hashem told Jacob, "I will guard you wherever you go," it was prudent for Jacob not to put himself or his family in harm's way.

The second danger was if Esau did not wage war and tried to be nice to him. Esau offered to escort Jacob and Jacob begged off. Jacob was concerned about the risks of maintaining a relationship with Esau. He knew, from his dealings with Lavan, that it was highly unlikely that a positive, continuing relationship could develop. Good things from bad people are not such good things. The apparent loving and caring behavior from an evil person is just a ploy to control and eventually overpower the other.

It was best that they parted. We saw that Jacob and Lavan each went their own way. Jacob and Esau parted and continued their individual travels.

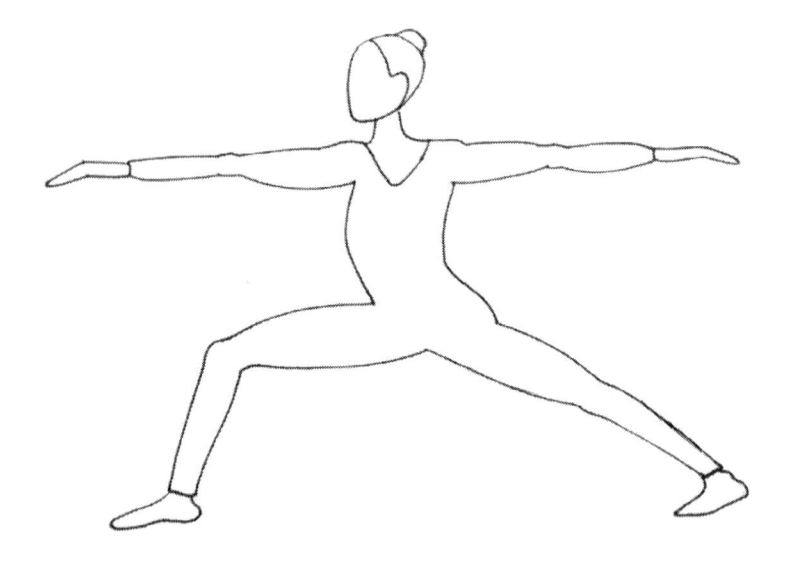

Yoga—Warrior pose arms out

Standing with your legs apart as wide as comfortable.
Arms out.
Turn both feet left.
Look over your left arm.
Bend your left leg at knee.
Sink into position.
Breathe and hold pose.
Straighten left leg and come up.
Turn both feet forward.
Now, turn both feet to the right.
Arms out.
Look over your right arm.
Bend right leg at knee.
Sink into position.
Breathe and hold pose.
Straighten right leg and come up.

Vayeishev (and he settled)

Parsha Insight — All I want is peace

All I Want is Peace
"Jacob settled in the land of his father" after his many years of being away. He spent fourteen years studying in the yeshiva of Shem and Eber, twenty years living with Lavan and now he wanted to settle and live his life in peace.

We saw Jacob growing from the studious, quiet son to the patriarch of a large family. We saw his development into a smart and discerning man who learned how to deal with the evil people in this world. Now, in his senior years, he wanted to live a peaceful life.

Is This a Problem?
Jacob was not wanting to lie back, relax and have a piña colada. He had already achieved a level of growth and completeness. "Jacob arrived intact (whole, perfect) at the city of Shechem (in Israel)" (Vayishlach 33:18). He now wanted to devote himself to the service of God.

Too much comfort, too much peace and too much security make one complacent, and these become obstacles rather than benefits. Think about a job we had or presently have. At first it was a challenge and we stretched ourselves to do well. We were excited about each day and looked forward to further growth and opportunities to excel. We became proficient and accomplished, and it became easy to keep this level of achievement. It went from easy to boring. Boring became no challenge and no challenge became room for negative activities. We wasted time, we weren't as careful, we took chances and basically our production suffered. We are programmed to need a challenge, perhaps a little bit of tumult, to keep the thoughts and effort flowing.

Discord Among the Brothers

Joseph told his brothers about his dream of all of them gathering sheaves and their bundles bowing down to his bundle. He told his family the dream about the sun and the moon and the stars bowing down to him. The brothers thought that Joseph was dreaming about usurping them and becoming the only continuation from Abraham, Isaac and Jacob, the Avos who were selected to continue the Jewish people while their siblings were not. Jacob's sons were angry and jealous that Joseph's progeny might possibly become the only continuation of Abraham's legacy.

Joseph was seventeen at the time and a very handsome youth. Perhaps he was a little full of himself. Youth is impetuous and says things without thinking them through. If Joseph had listened to his own words, he would have realized that he was provoking a negative response. Joseph knew that these dreams were a prophecy and that they would instill jealousy in his brothers. Even his father scolded him when Joseph told him the dreams. Rashi says that Jacob took the dreams seriously and scolded Joseph so that his brothers would not resent him.

Free Will

Reuben told his brothers not to shed Joseph's blood. Instead of killing him, they put him in an empty pit. The pit was empty of water but there were scorpions and snakes in the pit. Reuben's reasoning was that humans have free will but animals do not. If the brothers mortally wounded Joseph, they would be using their free will. If the scorpions and snakes killed Joseph, it would be an act of God. Animals don't have free will, they act upon God's orders. Falling into the hands of humans with free will is more dangerous than being in harm's way with animals. Reuben knew that Hashem's mercy would protect Joseph.

Pillar of Torah
Ramban said, "An important principle and a pillar of all Torah and mitzvahs" is free will. Each person makes his own choice whether to be good or to be evil. If every action was preprogrammed, how could you punish one for his sins or reward one for his mitzvahs? The Ramban placed responsibility upon the individual. We can be blamed if we choose to do evil. When we use our characteristics and choose to do mitzvahs, we merit reward. The greatest reward is in meeting our potential and perfecting ourselves in the service of Hashem.

Joseph's Story Continues
Joseph was taken from the pit by traders and traded several times until he wound up in Egypt as a slave. His master's wife tried to seduce him and he was wrongly jailed. While in jail he befriended two other prisoners, the Pharaoh's baker and his wine steward, and interpreted their dreams. When the wine steward was about to be released from prison, Joseph made him promise to mention to Pharaoh that he was still imprisoned and ask for his release. He asked twice. The parsha ends with the words, "Yet the Chamberlain of the Cupbearers did not remember Joseph, but he forgot him."

Yoga—Child's pose for all Jacob's children

All of Jacob's children built the Jewish Nation and formed the twelve tribes.

Start in tabletop position.
Lean back toward your feet.
Hips are pressing down towards your heels.

Open child's pose is with knees spread out to mat edge and arms extended forward.
Closed child's pose is with knees together and arms at your sides.
Find the pose that is most comfortable for you.
This is a good resting pose.

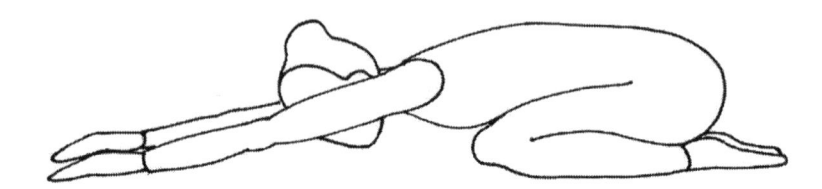

Mikeitz (and in the end)

Parsha Insight—What's the rush?

Don't Ask Twice
We pick up the story of Joseph languishing in prison an additional two years because he asked the wine steward twice to remember him to Pharaoh. Why was he punished? If I ask my son to buy me a container of milk before he comes to my house, and then tell him, "Now, don't forget the milk," will I be punished with not being able to have milk for two years? Probably not. My son has a habit of forgetting and I'm not a great tzaddik. A tzaddik is a righteous person very learned in Torah.

Tzaddik Status
What does tzaddik status have to do with asking for something two times? Joseph was a tzaddik and the friendship with the wine steward was created by Hashem to assist Joseph's release from prison. Joseph trusted in Hashem but it seems that his bitachon only went so far. Not far enough to trust that he would be remembered and released. Wait a minute! He did trust Hashem, it was the wine steward who he feared would not remember him.

This explanation is from Rabbeinu Bachya, whose full name is Bahya ben Joseph ibn Paquda. He lived in Spain during the first half of the eleventh century. In his *Guide to the Duties of the Heart* he says that Joseph saw God's hand as paving the way for his release from prison. His level of learning and understanding holds him to a higher degree than me or you. We can ask twice that our son remember the milk and the only consequence might be our son saying, "Yeah, Mom, I heard you." For Joseph, the tzaddik, asking once was proper hishtadlus (doing his job) and asking twice was not proper bitachon (trust in God).

And in the End
Two years (to the day) went by and Pharaoh had a bad dream. He called in his wise men, including the wine steward, who suddenly remembered Joseph and his ability to interpret dreams. This immediately got Joseph released from prison and he gave a brilliant explanation of the dream of seven good years and seven lean years. Joseph was promoted to viceroy, second in command of Egypt.

God had a plan all along. The Chazon Ish, Avrohom Yeshaya Karelitz (1878-1953), says, "The true description of bitachon is the belief that there is no coincidence in this world and that everything that transpires occurs with Hashem's approval and instructions."

Why the Rush?
"It happened at the end of two years (to the day)" and Joseph was rushed from the dungeon. In the Stone Chumash, "incidents of Divine salvation come hastily and unexpectedly" (p. 224, note 14).

When something is supposed to occur there is no time wasted. A window of opportunity opens and it behooves us to act upon it. We can almost feel the "rush" that propels us along. It seems as if the matter is taken out of our hands and that Hashem is doing the work.

Wasting Time
Are you guilty of these time wasters? (from Success Magazine)

Time Wasters
Talking too long on the phone or too much TV time.
Too frequently browsing social media sites.
Incessantly preparing and not taking action.
Failing to say no to unrelated tasks.
Failing to ask for help or follow directions.
Waiting until late in the day to do tasks.
Having a disorganized office or house.
Focusing on smaller, less important tasks.

Controlling Your Time
Set a time limit for non-task-related Internet browsing.
Plan out the most pressing task and break it up into manageable sections.
Make a short daily to-do list and say no to tasks not on that list.
Set deadlines and alarms for you to complete tasks.
Do the quick, short jobs first.
Stop procrastinating NOW.

Yoga—Standing plank pose

Pushing too much to make something happen usually does not work in our favor.
Make the effort, do what can be done, and know when it is enough.

When pushing is okay
The traditional plank pose is on the ground and you push yourself up by your arms like a push-up.
This is a gentler plank pose.
We will do our plank pose using the wall.
Stand about twelve to eighteen inches away from the wall.
Put your palms flat on the wall.
Your arms are at shoulder height.
Lean towards the wall so that your head is at the wall.
Your body is at an angle but not bent.
Push your palms into the wall.
Push hard and at the same time bring your body straight.
Your feet have not moved.

Vayigash (and he drew near)

Parsha Insight—Strength

Brilliant Speech
Joseph was viceroy of Egypt. His brothers had come to obtain food because there was a famine in Canaan. He recognized them, but they did not recognize him. He wanted to see whether they had changed since they had sold him into slavery, so he had some of his belongings hidden in Binyamin's possessions. His soldiers "found" them there and brought the brothers back. Our parsha begins at this point, when Yehuda pleads with Joseph.

Yehuda's speech to Joseph is brilliant and he shows himself to be the true leader of the brothers. Perhaps that is why we are called Yehudim.

Yehuda approaches Joseph and begins, "If you please, my lord," very politely and respectfully. He then asks if he could speak in Joseph's ears. He wants permission to speak bluntly and he wants Joseph to really listen: not just to hear the words but to look deeply into the words. He requests that Joseph "not let his anger flare up." "You are like Pharaoh," he says, referencing Joseph's position, strength and, perhaps, hardness of heart. Yehuda retells the entire saga, including the death of one son (Joseph), adds some embellishments, and speaks about his father's age and love for his youngest son, Binyamin.

I Am Joseph
Joseph orders everyone out of the room except the brothers, and he cries out, "I am Joseph. Is my father still alive?" This is a rhetorical question and a rebuke for what the brothers had done to him. In other, less eloquent and much blunter words: you weren't so worried about our father when you captured me and had me sold into slavery. How can you carry on about your father over Binyamin? Jacob survived my disappearance.

The key purpose of any reproof should be to get the person to understand the wrongs that he did. It is not to criticize or embarrass. Joseph's statement is powerful. It is simple and it makes the point exquisitely. "But his brothers could not answer him because they were left disconcerted before him." Joseph saw his brothers' shame and their understanding of his rebuke, and went to them lovingly and said, "It is me." He told them not be distressed and not to reproach themselves, and to know that it was God's will that sent him to Egypt before them so that they would survive the famine.

When we give our children reproof we need to follow up with loving ways. Little children need boundaries and need to be reprimanded for unbecoming behavior. They also need to see your love and know that their actions may be unloving but they are not.

This is not any different with adult children. We watch them conduct their lives and don't want to interfere. But sometimes we need to express our opinions. Why do we feel such an urgent need to tell them what we think? Am I still trying to set the boundaries for my children? Am I trying to mold them into replicas of me? Do I have the answers as to how they should live?

I've thought about this a lot and found that when my children do something that I don't approve of, I just want to help them make their lives easier. Most of the things they are going through, I experienced. I want them to learn without some of the pain. We can learn from Joseph. Say something, ONCE, in a short concise statement and then show love and respect.

The brothers returned to Israel with riches from Egypt and prepared to transport Jacob and all their families to Egypt. At first Jacob could not believe that Joseph was alive. Once he heard the whole story he said, "How great! My son Joseph still lives! I shall go and see him before I die." Jacob's spirit was revived.

The Days and the Years

Pharaoh and Jacob meet. Jacob appears frail and very aged. He is presented by Joseph. Presented? That brings an image to mind of Jacob holding on to his son, Joseph. Jacob blesses Pharaoh and these two great men talk to each other. Pharaoh asks Jacob, "How many are the days of the years of your life?" What is the reason to ask about the days of the years? The days refer to days of truly living and the years refer to chronological age. Jacob replies that he is not as old as his forefathers. That the truly good days of his life are few and that his forefathers had more days of living.

Jacob has just told Pharaoh that he had a hard life. It showed on his face and in his posture. The way we see ourselves is how we present ourselves to others. Pharaoh was astute and recognized the difference between living and being alive.

Are we truly living our days or are we just spending time alive? Hashem has given us everything we need to live full and productive lives. We just have to look at ourselves and see our resources. Most of us recognize what we have, our families, our jobs, the house, the car, the bank account. Are we fully aware of all our inner resources? It is said that when trouble comes, we have available all kinds of inner strength to deal with the issues. Don't wait for trouble. Harvest all the strengths that Hashem gave you. Do it now! This is the time to become the best you that you can be. All improvements, all learning, all changes are done in this world, before we pass to the next. Don't waste this opportunity. To live each day is to recognize your potential, to be happy with the strengths that you have, and to use them.

Jacob looked old. Our attitudes show on our face and in our posture. A healthy mind helps your body to be healthy. A psychosomatic disease affects both the mind and the body. Stress and anxiety can make a physical problem worse. We can understand how being nervous and full of anxiety could increase blood pressure, cause a rash and bring on ulcers.

Yoga—Mountain pose

We aim for a healthy mind and a healthy body.
According to the Mayo Clinic website, "Yoga is a mind-body practice that combines stretching exercises, controlled breathing and relaxation. Yoga can help reduce stress."
"Yoga brings together physical and mental disciplines to achieve peacefulness of body and mind, helping you relax and manage stress and anxiety."
"Hatha yoga is a good choice for stress management. Beginners like its slower pace and easier movements. Almost anyone can do it."

Strong pose bringing together physical strength and discipline of mind.
Standing tall.
Feet together.
Raise your arms straight up over your head.

Breathe slowly, in and out through your nose.
This is a position of strength and balance.

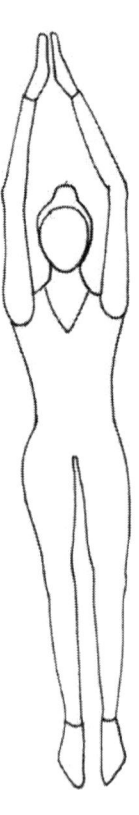

Vayechi (and he lived)

Parsha Insight — How we see our lives

The Gematria of Vayechi is Thirty-Four
Jacob tells Joseph that he lived seventeen years in Egypt — the years after his reunion with Joseph — and the seventeen years from Joseph's birth. So Jacob lived thirty-four years; the rest of his years he saw as a troubled existence. In the last parsha, Pharaoh asked Jacob, "How old are you?" He asked because when he looked at Jacob's face, he looked old, he looked tired, he looked beaten down. Jacob said, "I had a hard life." Now Jacob is saying that he only lived the seventeen years in Egypt and the seventeen years that Joseph lived with him before being taken away by his brothers.

The gematria of vayeichi is thirty-four and is based on the numerical value of the letters of the word vayeichi.

Our Life is How We Interpret It
Each of us is given a separate and unique life. Each life is one of a kind. Our nature and nurture, packaged with our predispositions, are individual. We each have situations that enable us to grow and to be challenged. This is our opportunity to use our free choice, to use the wisdom, the insight and the discernment we have been given by Hashem.

Jacob looked at his life and said that he had a hard life. That was his choice. Our job is to be the best that we can be, given the life setting that we have. Our life is unique and created so that we can bring out the best in us. It is often said that where you have the most trouble is where you need the most work.

If you look back and you have always had trouble with income, you need to reflect and see what you could do differently. What you could do to change the way things occur. What you could do to improve your financial situation. Although we have faith in God and trust that God is active in our lives, we still have to do our part to make the effort to improve our lives and to make the right choices.

We each have a "story" that we tell ourselves about our lives. Check out your story. Write down your description of your life. Read it over and see if you come away with a positive or negative image of your past. Did you highlight all the setbacks you had? Is your story filled with your accomplishments? WYSIWYG. What you see is what you get!
Just in case you read ahead to this paragraph and had decided to write only good things, if it was a "fight" not to bemoan the divorce, the job loss, the bad decisions, and so on, know that you have some work to do. The past is set and you can't change it.

What you can do is reframe the situations. This means that you look at the event and see what occurred because it happened. For example, your job was phased out and you found yourself unemployed. This propelled you into a new career that you are thoroughly enjoying and making good money. Another example, your adult children move to another community, far away from you. One is in Israel, one in California and the other lives in New Jersey. Look at all the places you now can visit and see the kids.

We can go on. You get the message. Your life is how you see it. The events will occur with Hashem's will. We have the free choice to see them as a positive or negative thing. Make God's will my will, so that my will is God's will.

The Awe of Hashem
When Jacob knew that Joseph was coming to visit him when he was sick, and bringing his two grandsons, Jacob made the effort to sit up for the visit. Rashi says that this is Jacob showing respect for the king. Joseph at this time was second in command behind the Pharaoh in Egypt. Jacob showing respect for the king, showing respect for his son and his grandchildren, is as we show respect to Hashem.

I remember visiting my father when he was sick. He had a series of strokes and was in the hospital. His right side was affected, as was his speech. It was very difficult for me and I could see that it was hard for my father. I saw that he did not want me to see the frozen look on his face where the muscles weren't working anymore. He didn't want me to see the hand that wasn't moving anymore. He took the covers with his left hand to cover the damaged right hand. He didn't want to frighten me. At that time I was a forty-year-old woman. I was not a child. Still, my father did not want me to see that he was not the strong man of my childhood. My father was showing respect for his adult child.

I was sick when my children were young. My son was ten and my daughter was thirteen. I was very concerned that because I was ill my children would be frightened and they would have questions that they would not ask because of their fear. I wanted to sit up, have my hair combed, and be wearing a nice nightgown when they saw me. I wanted to look good so they would feel okay — they would be comforted. I was showing respect for my young children.
It is a mitzvah to visit a sick person, and when you visit, you take away 1/60th of the sickness. May we all be blessed with sixty visitors if we are sick.

Yoga—Bridge

Our yoga practice will follow the theme of each of us being created differently, each of us in a setting that is unique to us. Our pose will be the bridge pose. There are all different kinds of bridges—long ones and short ones, high ones and low ones. Your bridge pose will represent where you are today in your yoga practice.

Lie on the floor with your feet flat on the floor and your knees up, hip-width apart.
Hands, palms down on the floor.
Using your hands and your feet for support, press your torso up.
Your head and your shoulders remain on the floor.
Hold your bridge pose for five long and deep inhales and exhales, if you can.

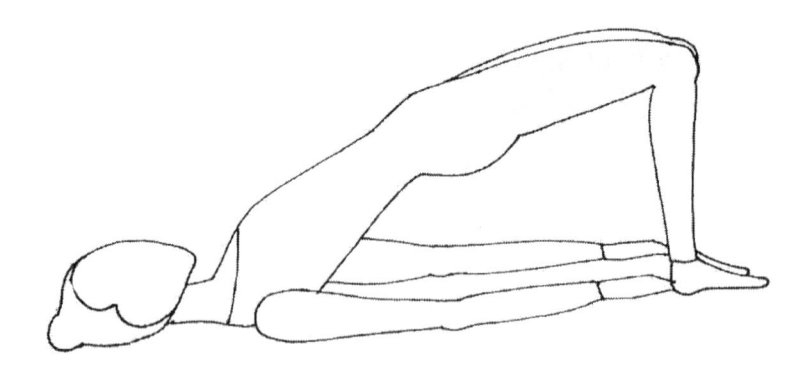

Book II

Shemos/Exodus

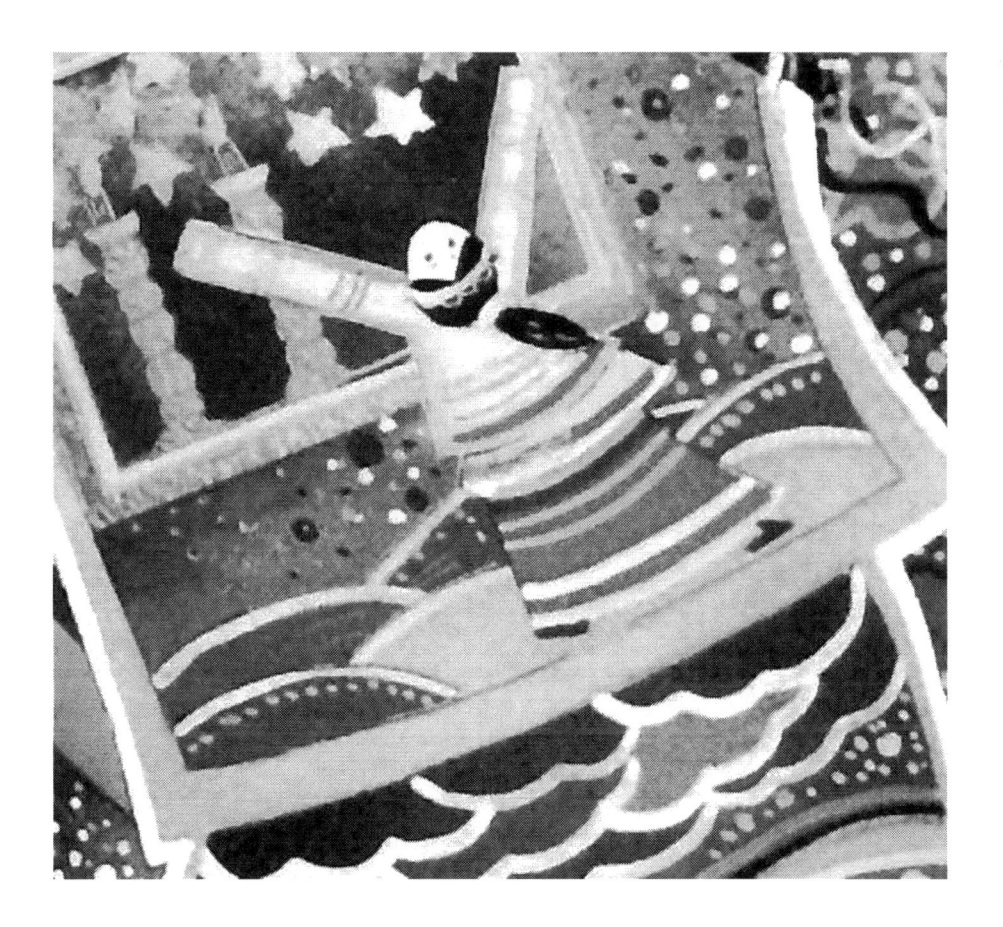

Shemos (names)

Parsha Insight — Decline

We Each Count
The Torah lists all the names of the Children of Israel who came with Jacob to Egypt. Why is the Torah repeating itself?

Rashi, a major commentator on Chumash, and his p'shat (simple) interpretations that have the most direct meaning, cites "Midrash Tanchuma." Rashi says that Hashem named all the people this second time because it was very important that we had each person by name and not just by number.

Everybody is an individual. We have said that each person has a set of circumstances and situations that are unique to him, and that each of us is different from any other person. We look different and act different and have our individual identity. Rashi is saying that it takes each and every one of us to make klal Yisroel, the people of Israel. If one of us is missing, we are not complete. We each count.

Proud Jew to Oppressed Slave
The change from a proud people, with each person's own individuality, coming to Egypt and then the decline to bondage happened after all of Joseph's brothers died. Pharaoh respected Jacob and he depended upon and appreciated Joseph and his brothers. By the time all the brothers were dead, decrees were put in place that were taking the Jews from individuality to bondage. These decrees started with taxes that grew more onerous. If you could not pay off your tax debt, you did not go to debtor's prison. You became a slave to work off your debt. The slave work was oppressive. It was not work that you could be proud of doing, it was not work in which you could see any accomplishment. The parsha takes us from the proud Jew to the oppressed slave.

Hashem had decreed that the Jews would be oppressed, subjugated to bondage in a strange land, a foreign land. We know that the Egyptians were punished for doing this. Since Hashem had decreed this, couldn't the Egyptians say that they were just carrying out Hashem's decree? So why were the Egyptians punished?

Well, for one, they opted for the job; and two, they were harsh beyond need. They did not have to be mean and hateful. The beatings, the oppressive labor, the cruelty were not necessary. When Moses came to Pharaoh and asked him to release the Jews, Pharaoh did not release them. He made the slavery even crueler.

Parable
Sam was supposed to die on a certain day. On that day, Len came and killed Sam. Is Len exonerated for Sam's murder because the death was decreed by Hashem? The answer is no, because who told Len to make the freewill choice to do the job? Sam could have died in any number of ways. Len took it upon himself to murder Sam. We are responsible for our actions; so, too, the Egyptians were responsible for their actions.

Yoga—Mountain pose, swan dive, deep forward bend

The yoga pose will start with an upright position to represent the proud Jews who came into Egypt. Then we will dive down to signify the deep and intense decline into bondage, where we find the Jews at the end of the parsha.

Mountain pose
Standing tall, proud, straight,

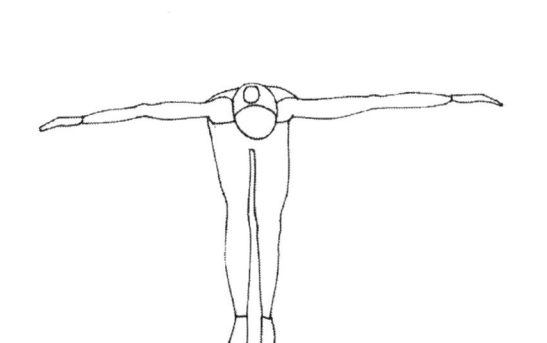

bring your arms up over your head.

Now swan dive
Arms outward in wide circle.

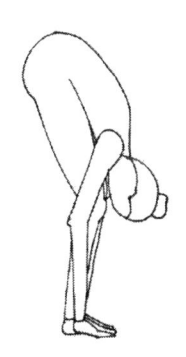

Deep forward bend.
You can bend your knees.
Your head reaches down towards the ground.
Your arms are heavy.

Vaeira (and I appeared)

Parsha Insight—Realize your potential

There Are Many Different Names for God
God (Elohim) spoke to Moses and said to him, "I am Hashem" (Adonoy). Elohim means justice and Adonoy means mercy. These different names represent two different attributes of God that are brought out in this opening sentence of the parsha.

Justice versus Mercy
What is God saying to Moses? He is talking about justice in contrast to mercy. Justice is judgment. God could have invoked justice as a rebuke for the complaining that Moses had done: "I can't do it. I don't speak well enough. The people are not going to listen to me." It was a reprimand to Moses for the doubts that he had about his role of representing Hashem to the Children of Israel. But Adonoy is merciful. Justice by itself would be too harsh if there wasn't any mercy, feeling sorry, taking pity and understanding. Judgment is tempered by deferment, severity and teshuva.

Justice is moderated by deferring punishment. There are many bad people who do miserable things, yet they don't die instantly. This is a deferred punishment. They will get theirs in time to come, but not right this minute.

Judgment can be tempered by the reduction of the severity of the lesson. Each of the lessons of our lives has a measured severity. The less severe judgment is tempered by mercy.

Another temperament of judgment is teshuva, repentance. If we recognize our errors, ask forgiveness and make every effort not to repeat the errors, we are doing teshuva and judgment is lessened with mercy. A complete teshuva is when we know that we will not repeat the errors of our ways. A wonderful example of Hashem's mercy is giving us the gift of teshuva.

We Resist Change
Later on in the parsha it says, "Adonoy spoke to Moses and Aaron," using the name Adonoy, mercy. God told them to take the Children of Israel out of Egypt. Moses was concerned that the Children of Israel would not listen because of shortness of breath and hard work. They had so much onerous work that their minds could not relate to being taken out of Egypt. "Shortness of breath" means that they were familiar with the idols of Egypt and it would be a hardship to leave them. Nobody likes to make changes. Even when the change is going to be a good one, we still resist change. Moses had to teach the Jews how to live without idols. Moses had to teach them in a merciful way and that is by doing it slowly. Complete and drastic changes are not welcome and are resisted. A gradual change gives one time to get used to it little by little before moving on to another stage.

Basic Job of a Person
When Hashem spoke to Moses and Aaron, sometimes He said Moses and Aaron and sometimes He said Aaron and Moses. This tells us that both brothers were equal. Each had to do the tasks they were given using their God-given attributes. Anyone who fully uses his talents is a great person. We are not measured by how many things we accumulate, how much money we have, how many vacations we go on or how many parties we attend. We are measured by the percentage of our God-given talents that we have taken advantage of, those we have developed and from which we have grown the most. Our basic job in this world is to improve our characteristics, traits and skills and not leave any potential undeveloped.

My bundle of characteristics is different from anybody else's package. No two people are alike. This is so empowering. Each of us is individual and has all the skills necessary to do the tasks before us. It takes away all matters of "I don't have enough, I wish I had this or that." Rather, we each have what we need to do what we have to do. We get the package that Hashem wanted for us and we get it with all the raw materials we need. Our job is to bring it to fruition, to its full potential. We need to put aside anything that is thwarting us from reaching this full potential. We can't be sidetracked or lulled into passiveness.

How will we be measured? We will be measured by the percentage of potential we have developed. What a shame to see our life in retrospect and realize all that we have not mastered. All the things we could have done, but never tried because of fear. Goals that were within our province that we just did not attempt.

Yoga—Shoulder stand and plow

I have a very hard pose so that we can aim to realize our potential in our yoga practice. It is a shoulder stand and plow pose. It takes practice.
This is a difficult pose. If you are a beginner, talk to your physician about your exercise program and do not do difficult poses before you are ready.

Shoulder stand
Start by lying on your back with your legs up the wall.
Your rear is at the right angle of the wall and the floor.
Your legs are straight up.
Put your hands under your rear and walk your feet up the wall.
You are supporting yourself on your shoulders.
Your legs are straight up in the air.
Balance.

Plow
Now fold and lower your legs towards your head. Keep your legs straight. Your arms are palms down on the ground.

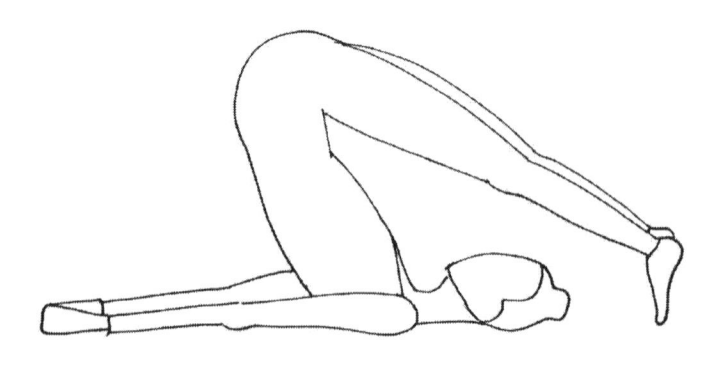

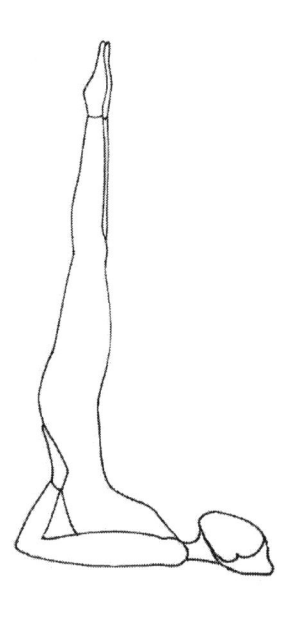

Bo (enter)

Parsha Insight — Darkness

The Ten Plagues
The seven plagues in the last parsha, Vaeira, in order, are: blood, frogs, lice, wild beasts, epidemic, boils and hail.

Hashem hardened Pharaoh's heart with the seventh plague. Before the plague of hail, Pharaoh had free will and could choose his actions. The seventh plague in parsha Vaeira was hail, a very special hail with fire inside. The eighth plague was locusts. There were so many of them that they were stacked up. People had to push them away to walk through them. The ninth plague was darkness and that is the subject of this chapter. The tenth plague was death of the firstborn.

The plague of darkness differs from the previous eight plagues. The locusts and the frogs were bad in a simple manner. However, darkness suggests a moral darkness, an internal darkness. We sometimes say "a darkness came over him." We don't mean that there wasn't any light. We are saying that he is mired in his evil. He lost moral standing.

Did Hashem Have a Sense of Humor?
Think about the Passover Seder. In many homes, on the second Seder night the kids are throwing plastic frogs and marshmallows. There is something humorous about the plagues. They are absurd. Was Hashem playing with the Egyptians with the plagues? By the time we get to the ninth plague, if there is humor it seems dark (pun intended). The greatest of the Egyptian gods is Ra, the sun god. The plague of darkness has no sun, no light. Ra is ineffective. Hashem's strength is shown.

Not an Ordinary Darkness

This darkness was not an ordinary darkness. This was a darkness with a deep meaning. Hashem created the world with utterances and He created light. Hashem did not create darkness; it is simply what there is without light. The darkness of the ninth plague was not only an absence of light. It was a different and separate kind of darkness. It was a darkness that had a thickness to it. It was thick enough that people could not make their way through it. With the locusts, there were so many that the people had to push their way through them. They could not push through this darkness. The people were immobilized by the darkness so that the position in which the darkness found them was the position in which they stayed.

When we think of darkness we assume blackness. We can't see; maybe we imagine evil. Not only can't we see form and figure, we can't see truth. There is no light of Torah. We are stuck in the darkness. We use this in speech as a way to explain how we might be trapped in ourselves, that we have a darkness in our heart. While the Egyptians experienced this darkness, the Jews did not. The Jews had light; they were able to see. The knowledge of Torah is the light of Torah.

Promptness and Timing

This is an intense darkness. This darkness is a warning to the Jews, who were at the forty-ninth level of their descent into the fifty levels of degradation. They were almost lost completely, but they still had light. The Jews still had a chance to redeem themselves. When it was time to leave Egypt, it was time to leave at that precise moment; not before and not a second after. If the Jews had not left at the precise time, all would have been lost.

Leaving Egypt was a spiritual event and the timing is spiritual. Just as creation occurred with God's utterances, the moment of Joseph's release from prison, and the Jews leaving Egypt, all had to happen at the precise moment. These were not natural events, they were events created by God according to His plan. The Jewish Nation was being created as we stood at the forty-ninth level of descent.

In Parsha Bo it says, "Guard the matzos." Matzos have to bake for eighteen minutes, not more and not less. Guarding the matzos is a reference to promptness and timing: the right time for the Jews to leave Egypt.

Yoga—Balance pose

Darkness changes our balance.
Darkness takes away your stability.
Nothing else changes but closing our eyes.

Stand with both legs together.
Put the right foot in front of the left foot and keep your hands on your hips.
This is a balance pose.
Focus on an unmovable point to keep your balance.
Now close your eyes. Not so easy.

Do the same thing with the left foot in front of the right foot.

Bishalach (when he let go)

Parsha Insight — Reactions to adversity

The parsha opens with Moses and all the Jews who left Egypt with him at the banks of the Yam Suf or the Red Sea (Sea of Reeds). The Egyptians are bearing down on them. What is their response?

Four Courses of Action
Moses conveys Hashem's message "Stand fast. Hashem will do battle on your behalf. You shall not see the Egyptians like this again. Remain silent."

Moses is speaking to four groups of people, each of which has a different response to the situation.

Group One says, "Let's just jump in the water and die."
Group Two says, "Let's do battle with the Egyptians."
Group Three says, "Let's go back to Egypt."
The fourth group says, "Let's yell and scream and carry on and make a lot of confusion."

Assurances
"Stand fast" and see what Hashem will do. Don't jump into the water and die.
"Hashem will do battle on your behalf." Don't battle the Egyptians. Hashem will do the battles; you don't have to.
"You shall not see the Egyptians like this again." Don't go back to Egypt as slaves. You are not going to see Egyptians ever again from this weakened position.
"Remain silent." What's with the noise and the screaming? Be quiet.

Trust in Hashem
Manna, food, falls from heaven. Trust in Hashem is needed because the people only get a daily portion; manna that is hoarded over week nights spoils by morning. Also, no manna can be gathered on Shabbos. It is necessary each night to trust that in the morning there will be food available for the day and a double portion on Friday for Shabbos. The Shabbos portion remains fresh and usable.

While the Temple stood in Jerusalem, two showbreads were placed on the altar each Shabbos to symbolize the double portion of manna that fell on Friday; and to this day, two challahs — braided Sabbath bread — are put on the Sabbath table for the Friday night and Saturday noon meals.

Major Lessons
When we have a problem, what do we do? How do we handle a difficulty? Do we make a lot of noise and scream and yell; go back to our prior position; make a huge fight; or give up and say, "Crawl all over me, I'm just a doormat anyway?"

Most of us use one of these four options when we have a problem. We think we are in total control. Making a quick decision is not using patience and trust. This doesn't mean that we should do nothing and wait for Hashem to save us. It means that sometimes the quick, first reaction is not the way to go. The story might not be over yet. More information may be coming. We may not have to make that decision right now.

We start taking quick actions when we get impatient. When we lose our comfort level that things will happen, that others will act, that events will come about, we feel compelled to act. It is a lack of trust and patience. This comes from wanting to control and make things happen.

We really have to look at the whole situation, evaluate all our options, and come up with plans and actions that will make the most sense. We have to learn to balance emuna—faith—and hishtadlus—personal effort; to fine-tune our trust in God and to take our personal action. Sometimes we think that if we keep pushing, we will control things and make them happen. But we need to pause and listen for Hashem's voice in our inner workings to find the right amount and the correct effort for the particular situation.

Yoga—Patience

Patience and the finesse of knowing when to act and when to let it be are our lessons for this week. Yoga gives you the skills to step away and process information.

Symptoms of impatience
Feeling like you are not getting enough air.
Muscles tightening up.
Nervous body motions.
Belly tightening.
Quick actions.
Knee-jerk reactions.

Yoga helps to increase patience
Relaxes your body.
Emotions are calmed.
Breathe deeply.
Slow your breath down.
Slow your mind down.
Slow your body down.

Sit on your mat.
Cross your legs.
Palms on your knees.
Breathe in and out slowly.
Sit here long enough until you are just itching to get up.

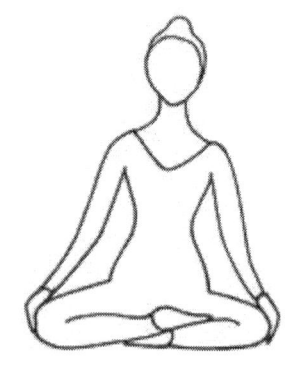

Yisro (abundance)

Parsha Insight — Really listen

Parsha Named for a Person
The name of the Parsha is Yisro, a person's name. In all the parshas, only six have someone's name. They are Noah, Sarah, Korach, Balak, Pinchas and Yisro. You would think that our forefathers, Abraham, Isaac, Jacob, Joseph, Moses and Aaron would merit having a Parsha named for them.

Listening is Not Only Hearing
Yisro, the father of Moses' wife, was a Midonite priest. Like everyone else, he heard about the splitting of the seas and the war with Amalek. Based upon these things, he — and he alone — decided to join the Israelites. He did not just hear the message, he listened to the message. The difference between hearing and listening is the comprehension and the internalizing of the message. When we say the Shema, we say "Hear Israel." The word shema means not just hearing with our ears, it means understanding and internalizing the message and making it ours. This means to actively listen to the message and take it to the next level. Yisro was able to do this while the rest of the population just heard the words but did not listen.

How to Really Listen
It is hard work to really listen when others are speaking. The first thing we have to do is stop thinking about what we are going to say as soon as he is quiet. Concentrate on the speaker. Look directly at the person talking. Do not fidget. We force ourselves to stop all judgments about the topic. We will have time later to interpret the meaning spoken. Do notice facial expressions and body language because they tell us much about the speaker's view of the topic. When it is time to ask questions, try to understand the speaker's position. Restate the speaker's words to be sure we understand what was said.

The Ten Commandments

The Ten Commandments are given in this parsha. The first thought is that the parsha should be named the Ten Commandments. This is big! But no; the parsha was named Yisro. This is because the comprehension of the message is as great as the message itself.

The world already had the seven Noahide Laws that are needed by people to live in society. If we kill people, steal from others, or seduce someone's wife, we cannot live in a community. Noahide Laws were given so that people would enjoy the world as humans instead of living like animals. These rules are acknowledged and automatically accepted just by being human. Built into our conscience and morality is a human soul that prevents us from functioning like dogs. Humanity was not given a choice about acceptance of the Noahide Laws.

These laws were named for Noah, the builder of the Ark that permitted his family and members of the animal kingdom of the world to survive the great flood that destroyed everything else. The Flood was brought about because the people had sunk so low that they were not fit to live in human society. They killed, fornicated without thought, did not care for their young, and took at will from others. There was no structure to society. Hashem needed to wipe the slate clean.

The Torah is Different

The Torah laws are not necessary to live in a human society. In fact, most of society does not live under Torah laws. So why did God give us the Torah? The Torah's positive and negative mitzvahs elevate us to a life of spiritual value. We go beyond the mundane existence of being simply a human in this world. A Torah life is about having the middos (the character traits) to function with honor and respect for others and for God. God gave the Torah; but like a package that is pointless until opened, the Torah had to be accepted.

Yoga—Tree pose, scales of justice

Yisro suggested that Moses appoint judges and develop a system of courts. The scales of justice are balanced with mercy. Let's do a balance pose for our yoga portion.

Put your weight on your right foot.
Lift your left foot to your ankle, shin, or upper thigh, not your knee.
Your arms are branches of the tree and may be up.
Now, hold your arms out with your palms up.
Justice is in one hand.
Mercy in the other.
Your hands on a straight line with each other.
Scales are balanced.
Justice and mercy balanced.

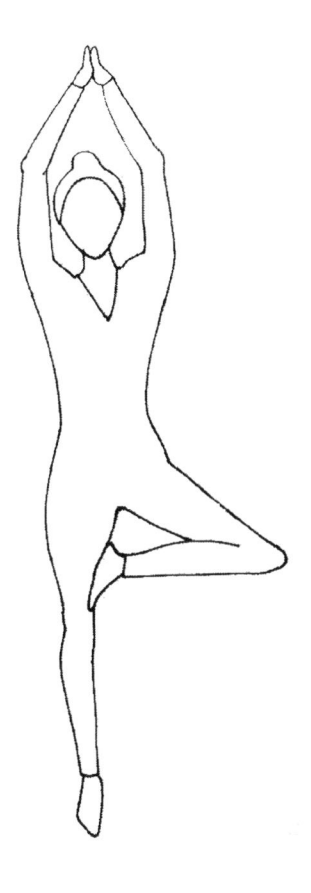

Mishpatim (judgments)

Parsha Insight—Tort and civil law

Continuation from Parsha Yisro
The seven Noahide Laws are basic human laws, applicable to all people. The Ten Commandments, which represent the synopsis of the 613 Mitzvahs, make humans mensches (moral, honorable people). Mishpatim means those laws that have a logical meaning and source.

In contrast, there are some mitzvahs in Torah that are called chukim. They have no logical meaning. Learned men have been able to ascribe some explanation to some of the chukim, for example, the mitzvah not to wear linen and wool in the same garment. Cain brought flax and Abel brought a sheep for offerings to Hashem. Hashem turned favorably to Abel but not to Cain. This caused jealousy and according to some is why we don't wear mixtures of linen and wool. Not really knowing if this is the reason for the mitzvah, it is called a chok.

This is My Favorite Parsha
Mishpatim are the laws that allow people to live together in a community. They are the basis for today's courts of tort and civil law.

The word mishpoche, which sounds so much like mishpatim, in Yiddish means "all the relatives." The mishpatim are the laws that relate to our dealing with others with law, order, justice and mercy. They are permanent laws, very much like secular laws in topic, except they are permanent. They are from God. It is not like the Bill of Rights, which can be amended.

Check Out Your Auto Insurance

These mishpatim are used today in courts of tort and civil law. All insurance contracts follow these laws of personal injury and property damage. I knew all these laws from my insurance career. Seeing them in Torah is amazing. This is where the laws originated. Just look at the auto insurance policy and see how it follows Torah. The contract conditions regarding bodily injury, property damage, medical payments, pain and suffering, and loss of ability to work are all in the insurance policy and all in Torah.

Laws of Property Damage

The laws of property damage came from the commandment not to steal. If I go to your house and sit with my mud-laden shoes all over your sofa, I will damage your furniture. How is this thievery? I have taken away from you the use of your property and caused you extra expense. I am prohibiting you from enjoying what you own. Thievery comes from a lack of emuna (faith), jealousy, coveting and being mean-spirited. I don't believe that Hashem will give me the means to take care of my needs, so I take them away from you. Hashem gave me all the resources I need to wipe my feet properly, but I'm either too lazy, too uncaring, or too selfish, so I steal value from you and use your sofa as a wipe cloth.

Or perhaps someone goes into your bathroom, sees your nice bracelet on the vanity and takes it. Negative middos prevail; coveting your belongings, stealing, dissatisfaction, not treating you with honor and respect, jealousy and meanness. The laws of property damage aim to financially restore people to where they were before the loss.

Sometimes we are guardians of another person's property. When I am in Florida, I give you the keys to my house and ask you to check it out every few days. You become a guardian. You can do this as a favor, for payment, or maybe you get some benefit out of being in my house. Perhaps I let you read my books. The laws are complicated; but the amount of benefit you derive determines the level of obligation that you have. The higher the benefit, the higher the level of responsibility. Total negligence bears responsibility. The Torah goes into all of this in explicit detail. In insurance and legal terms, we call the guardian the bailee and the owner the bailor.

Metaphor for Life
Why does the Torah go into the laws in such detail? They teach a person how to better serve Hashem. We have a body, mind and soul given to us by Hashem. We are the guardians of what was given to us and have a responsibility to use these resources in the proper manner and to be constantly vigilant to the blessings Hashem gives us. Our job is to protect, use and develop the resources we have and by doing this, we honor the trust that Hashem has in us.

If we misappropriate these resources, we are liable for it. These laws are a metaphor for us to guard our neshoma (soul) for Hashem. We have a total responsibility to protect our soul, our body and our minds.

What Does Torah Say About Exercise?
There is not much said about the need to exercise in the parshas. I don't think the Jews as slaves in Egypt needed to worry about getting enough exercise.

Maimonides writes, "A person should aim to maintain physical health and vigor, in order that their soul may be upright, in a condition to know God. For it is impossible for one to understand sciences and meditate upon them when he is hungry or sick, or when any of his limbs is aching." The Rambam defined exercise as "vigorous or gentle movement, or a combination of the two."

Yoga—Find a yoga routine

Hashem wants us to stay with our body as long as we can.
There is no more growth without the body.

Find a 20- to 30-minute (at least) yoga practice that will help you get in touch with your whole body.
It could be a flow in and out of many positions.
This will keep your body flexible and strong.
Try a gentle hatha yoga flow.
There are many audios of yoga practices.
Find one that you like. On the internet, most of the audios have a review function, which is very helpful in choosing the right one for you.

The Hatha yoga predominantly practiced in the West consists of mostly postures understood as physical exercises and accompanied with deep breathing. It is a stress-reducing practice.
This definition is from Wikipedia.

Terumah (offering)

Parsha Insight — Feel close to God

Do a Mitzvah with Enthusiasm and Diligence
When you have a mitzvah to do, follow instructions and do it with alacrity and zeal. Do not exhibit laziness or procrastination. Do the mitzvah with enthusiasm and diligence. It is so easy to say, "Well, it's 4 p.m., I can't do it today. I'm not as up for doing the mitzvah of visiting the sick in the late afternoon as in the morning. I'll do it tomorrow." In the upcoming parshas, jobs are being delegated and the people are responding to these tasks quickly and positively and not with apathy.

This parsha is about building the mishkan (the traveling tabernacle) and its utensils. This is building and creating the ark, the Temple, the menorah, the shulchan (table) and the sanctuary. Hashem says we are to make for Him a sanctuary so that He may dwell among us. Since God has no physical presence, is He subject to the boundaries of the mishkan? What is Hashem saying when He says that He will dwell among us?

Feel Close to Hashem
The mishkan is a place for us to gather to feel close to Hashem. We do not know what it was like to have the great Temple and have all Jews come together. We do know what it is like to come together in our eruv (neighborhood) and come together in shul (synagogue). We feel closer with Hashem in shul than we would if we were standing on the street. It is a place where we feel connected to Hashem. Hashem does not live in the shul and He didn't live in the mishkan as we "live" in our house. Perhaps when Hashem said, "I dwell among you," it means that Hashem resides in us. As we sanctify ourselves and our actions, perform mitzvahs and put holiness into the secular, these are examples of Hashem residing in us. And the sanctuary, the mishkan, alludes to our bringing Hashem into our lives.

The Tablets of the Law Were Carried

The Tablets of the Law were put in the ark and carried wherever the Jewish people went in the midbar, the desert. The ark had rings on the side and poles through the rings. Men would put the poles on their shoulders and walk with the ark. These poles remained in the rings and did not come out. The ark was always ready to move with the people.

Thirty-Nine Activities

The mishkan was built with thirty-nine basic occupations, and on the seventh day, nothing was created. Just as in Bereishis (Genesis), the seventh day was Shabbos and a rest day. These thirty-nine activities were stopped for Shabbos and have become the basis for what is and is not permitted to us on Shabbos. This gets complicated. To prevent us from accidentally doing forbidden activities on Shabbos, the rabbis have built a fence around them. They have decreed that related activities are forbidden so that we can't cross that line. We can do no sewing on Shabbos since sewing is one of the thirty-nine activities. The rabbis' fence around sewing means that the activity is expanded. A needle is muktzah—it can't be touched on Shabbos—and you can't put a needle into your lapel.

Symbolism of the Ark and the Utensils

The ark and the poles represent the partnership in Torah study of a learner and an earner. The partnership enables both to get benefit. The best-known partnership is of Zevulan and Issachar. Zevulan earned and Issachar studied Torah. Both doing their jobs properly gave each of them merit for both their own and their partner's effort. The ark and the poles of the ark remaining together are symbolic of this partnership for Torah study.

All of the mishkan and the utensils of the mishkan symbolize concepts and principles of Jewish life. The ark represents study of the written law. The shulchan is the table that held the showbreads. These showbreads remained fresh and warm from one Shabbos to another. At all times there were the two showbreads on the shulchan. This represents the sustenance of Jewish life. We trust that Hashem will give us what we need, just as we received two portions of manna on Friday so that we did not have to gather any on Shabbos.

The menorah represents the oral law and has three crowns: the Torah scholar, the Kohen and the King or man of wealth. All of these are nothing without the crown of a good name over it all. The menorah represents the practical fulfillment of the Torah — the everyday way of taking the secular and making it holy.

Betazel was given the task of building the mishkan and the utensils. He was a young man and did not have any previous construction experience or knowledge of any of the other occupations required for the mishkan. With faith that Hashem would show him how to do it, he became the master builder and general contractor.

Yoga—A special place to do yoga

I can't just flop down on the floor and do yoga. I need a set place and a set time with a level of quiet, an open view, and enough space so that I don't feel crowded. I can't have anything from outside coming into my space. Even an open closet door would make it difficult for me to do yoga. It would seem as though all the stuff in the closet was invading my space.

I am creating an environment, making a place where I can meet my yoga goals, not just doing the positions.

This is what the mishkan represented: a place where Hashem met us. When we left the mishkan we were filled with a sense of awe and gratefulness. After our yoga practice we leave our yoga space with a sense of peace and mindfulness.

Tetzaveh (you shall command)

Parsha Insight — Proper attire

Garments of the Kohanim
Very specific and exact details for each garment that is worn by the Kohen Gadol, the high priest, are given. These instructions are to be followed with no variations. The garments of each Kohen Gadol must be a perfect fit. The garments would not be appropriate if the shoulders were in the wrong spot, the sleeves too short, or the pants too long. A perfectly tailored garment creates a look and sense of being that is well-received. When the Kohen Gadol appears with garments that are well put together, he generates honor and respect.

The garments of the Kohen Gadol are called the bigdei kehuna. At the hem of the Kohen Gadol's outfit are bells and pomegranate-shaped cotton tassels. The bells make a tinkling noise and the cotton pomegranates are silent. Time for sound and time for quiet. We humans have speech and we have to use speech properly. "Improper speech" is not just bad words or bad ideas; sometimes it is our making noise when there should be quiet.

Proper Attire
The Jewish Nation is a kingdom of ministers. We dress properly, with our clothing showing dignity and decorum. Women wear modest clothing. Men cover their heads to show honor to Hashem. The attention to detail is important.

When we wear well-fitting and proper clothing it not only influences those who see us, it also influences how we see ourselves. Sometimes the outside does not match the inside. One can be very well-dressed and appropriate on the outside, but the inside does not match. When dealing with others, we have to discern the inside truth from what we see outside.

Breastplate
The choshen is the breastplate. It was worn by the Kohen Gadol over his heart to indicate that the inside middos, character traits, were as good as the outside appearance. In the breastplate was a parchment with Hashem's name. The breastplate had twelve semiprecious stones, one for each tribe. Each stone contained elements that related to the tribe to which it was ascribed.

Stones come from the earth and consist of minerals. They have healing properties. For example, amethyst is purple quartz, which is silicon dioxide. Its purple coloring is caused by iron or manganese compounds. Iron is a blood supplement and manganese is a bone supplement. The minerals of each of the stones can cure and heal something. When Hashem created a disease, He first made the cure. We have to catch up and find the cure.

Proper Speech
Before we say the standing prayer, the Shemoneh Esrei, we say "Open my lips that my mouth may declare your praise." We are asking God to let us speak and speak well, let honorable words come from our mouths. This parsha relates to loshon hora, improper speech. By not being quiet at the proper time and not speaking well, we engage in loshon hora. You are taking the gift of speech and turning it into something dirty. It is critical to watch our speech. Someone who watches his speech has a sense of self with humility. This is not being humble. It means knowing who you are and accepting yourself and properly using the gifts you were given.

Benjamin's stone was jasper; in Hebrew the name is yosh pei and pei is mouth. Jasper was for proper speech. One must be a true owner of his mouth and know when to use it and when to be quiet.

Yoga—Facial exercises, yoga clothing

We certainly are the owners of our mouths. So let's do a few yoga exercises to strength the muscles of our mouths and other facial features. Do each ten times.
Make mouth into small circle and then smile big, really big.
Put one finger into mouth, suck on it and pull out slowly.
Look straight ahead, pull neck skin down and lift head up.
Put your index fingers just above eyes and pull down and then raise eyebrows.
Put your fingers between the eyebrows, press the bump between eyes over nose, move eyebrows up and down.

Yoga clothing
The Kohen Gadol wore the proper clothing. Here are a few suggestions for proper yoga attire.
It is better to wear loose cotton clothing.
Tight elastic garments can be very restricting.
Wear pants or skirt with a loose elastic waist.
If you are wearing a skirt, be sure your movements are not confined.
Wear very stretchy leggings underneath the skirt.
If you wear a head covering, place any knot at the top and not at the back of the head. You should be comfortable when lying flat on the ground.

Ki Sisa (when you elevate)

Parsha Insight — Trust

Rich and Poor Alike
Each male over the age of twenty gave a half shekel for a census. Rich or poor, each gave the same amount, to show that each person counted regardless of their financial worth. There is no difference between the rich man and the poor man. Then the coins were counted. People were not counted because no person is a number.

Perspective of the Events
Days after leaving Egypt the people witnessed the destruction of the Egyptians at the Red Sea. The people sang the "Song of the Sea." Who is like you, God? They were overwhelmed at the majesty of Hashem and His saving them from the Egyptians.

In the third month after having left Egypt, they arrived at Mount Sinai and were given the Ten Commandments. There was thunder and lightning, and Hashem spoke the first two commandments to all the people. The people saw and trembled and stood from afar. They said to Moses, "You speak to us and we shall hear; let God not speak to us lest we die." It was too much for them to hear God's words directly. Moses was the intermediary between Hashem and the people.

Where's Moses?
Moses went up Mount Sinai to get the tablets with the Ten Commandments. He said that he would return on the fortieth day. By the people's count, the fortieth day had come and gone and Moses had not come back. This made the people very nervous. They were wondering what they would do if Moses did not come back. If Moses did not return, they would need a replacement. Otherwise they would have to speak to God directly, and they were afraid to do that.

Aaron's Role
They went to Aaron and said, "Rise up and make for us gods that will go before us." Aaron asked for gold. He thought the people wouldn't want to give it to him. But he was surprised how quickly the men were ready to give the gold to form an idol. Aaron took the gold and fashioned it into a molten calf, and he told the people that the next day they would have a festival for Hashem.

This was Aaron's way to soften the uprising. First, he put off the festival until the next day. He did not let the people pick another commander. He made sure that the people did not appoint him as their leader. Aaron was stalling for time. He knew that Moses would come back. He did not want the people, in their haste, to take actions that would create the problem of having to usurp a leader appointed in Moses' absence. The people looked at this golden calf as an intermediary between them and God, just as Moses was their intermediary with God.

What Moses Saw
The next day came and the festival got out of hand. The people were eating, drinking and reveling. They were giving elevation and peace offerings. Moses came down from Mount Sinai with the stone tablets with the Ten Commandments etched on them. He could not believe what he saw. Just forty days from the revelation, the people created an idol. Moses threw down the tablets and shattered them at the foot of the mountain.

Attributes of God
Moses said to Hashem, "Show me your ways." Hashem responded and revealed the thirteen attributes of God. "The Lord! The Lord! God, compassionate and gracious, slow to anger and abundant in kindness and truth, preserver of kindness for thousands of generations, Forgiver of iniquity, willful sin, and error, and who cleanses..." Moses asked Hashem to show him His glory; show him His essence. Hashem said, "You will see my back but not my face." We cannot know Hashem completely. The mysteries of God are not known by man; He is beyond human perception.

Lack of Trust
What happened with the people? Why did the people not trust that Moses would return? They were impatient, not calm, not serene, and not silent.

If I am using a shuttle service to the airport and my reservation has been confirmed, five minutes before the scheduled pickup I'm looking out the window, tapping my foot and getting nervous. Maybe I should call and check up on them. Maybe I should stand outside to make it quicker. It is so hard to just trust and give up control.

Yoga—Hold a position, knees to chest

Patience is such an important characteristic. Lack of patience makes us nervous and a bit irrational. Yoga gives us several positions that teach us to be more patient. The key is to tell yourself that you have no place else to be but where you are now. We get edgy and we become uncomfortable. Maimonides tells us to change a habit, take it to the other extreme so that we eventually come to a midpoint, a place of balance.

In this pose we shall push our patience to the point of uneasiness. We will soften the edge by concentrating on the yoga position and our breathing rather than thinking about where we need to be next.

Knees to chest
Lie on mat, flat on back.
Bring knees to chest.
Wrap your arms around your knees.
Grab each elbow with the other hand.
Don't force; if you can't grab your elbow, hold your knees.
Try to flex your feet.
Hold position for at least five complete breaths.
Breathe long and full inhales and exhales.
Release.

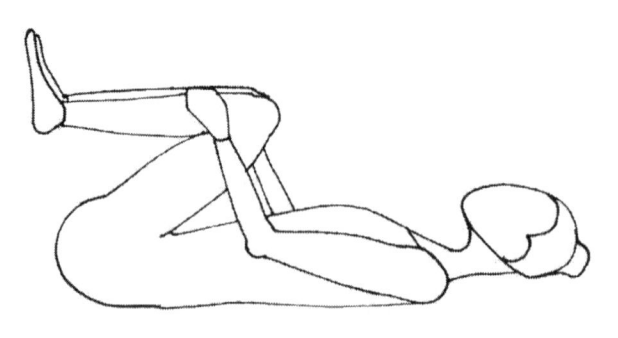

Vayakhel (and he assembled)
Pekudi (accountings of)

Parsha Insight — Free will

Shabbos
Moses gathered the Children of Israel together and told them, "You work for six days, but on the seventh day you stop all work. It is a holy day for you." The thirty-nine types of tasks, the melachas of creating the mishkan, are considered work in terms of the Sabbath. Briefly, these are: field work, sewing, leather fabrications, making the beams and the major construction pieces, kindling fire and the putting up and the taking down of the mishkan. The thirty-nine general categories of labor form the prohibitions of Shabbos.

Parsha Vayakhel opens with the laws of Shabbos. You can build the mishkan for six days but not on the seventh day. All work must cease, and we do not kindle any fires in our dwellings. This tells us that Shabbos takes precedence over holy work. Building the mishkan is holy work, but Shabbos is more holy. We don't kindle fires in our house because our home is our personal mishkan. Following these laws brings the holiness of the Shabbos into our home.

Rabbi Mendel Weinbach of Ohr Somayach said that the first mitzvah given to the Jewish people as a nation is the sanctification of the moon. Time is important and precious and, along with the beginning of a new month, Shabbos brings time into our consciousness.

Freewill Offering

Moses told everyone to bring a freewill offering to build the mishkan and create the utensils to be used in it. They are using their heartfelt donations to build the mishkan. This is not like the half-shekel donation that everyone must pay, rich or poor. This is a donation of what you can give, what you want to give, whether gold, silver, cloth or wood.

When they were in Egypt, the men were not particularly interested in their wives after a full day of hard labor. The women made themselves beautiful for their men and used their mirrors to check their appearance. The goal was to entice the men so that they could produce children and continue the Jewish people. Moses said at first, "No, do not bring mirrors to build the mishkan." He thought of the mirrors as symbols of vanity. But Hashem told him, "These women used the mirrors for a holy purpose, to grow the numbers of the Jewish people." So Moses accepted the mirrors.

Everything that was donated was used. The materials came from the people's hearts. Nothing would go to waste. When Moses saw that he was getting too many donations, he asked the people to stop. Miraculously, the craftsmen found a use for everything that had been donated up till that point. It was all used to make the mishkan and the utensils.

Exact Details

In parsha Pekudi the Torah goes into exact detail of how everything is to be made and the quantities of material to be used. Compare this detail to the sparse words in the previous parsha, Ki Sisa. When the women would not part with their gold for the golden calf, the men hurried up and gave their gold. Aaron took the gold, put it in the fire and fashioned it into a calf. One, two, three, golden calf. No details. It just became a golden calf.

Compare this to the mishkan and the utensils. Torah enumerates all the fine points of making the items and the loving attention to details.

When we follow Hashem's instructions, we make things holy. We take the secular and make it holy with mitzvahs. We do this to our homes and to ourselves. With Hashem in our lives, our body, mind, heart and soul are holy. Adhering to the details brings holiness to the mishkan, to our house and our bodies. We make ourselves holy with mindfulness.

When we pay attention and are mindful, we get added value to what is happening. We make the present moment meaningful and holy. What does holy mean? The Hebrew word, kadosh, that we translate into holy means set apart for a special purpose. Holy moments are set apart from all the rest of the goings-on, and therefore, special.

Choose to Belong
The book of Shemos takes the Jewish Nation from slavery to exile to revelation. The revelation is Hashem talking to us at the base of Mount Sinai. Jews must choose to belong. We need to make a freewill choice to be with the Jewish Nation.

Yoga—Pick your yoga

Choose the yoga practice that is right for you.
Here are just a few of the more popular types of yoga with only the basic focus itemized (from MatsMatsMats.com).

Bikram yoga
Comprehensive workout.
Muscle strength and endurance.
Cardiovascular.
Weight loss.
Yoga practice in a room with 95-105 degree temperature.

Chair yoga
Chair poses.
Promotes healing and transformation.
Good for senior citizens and persons with limited mobility.

Hatha yoga
Basic form of yoga.
Foundation of all yoga styles.
Poses and breathing.
Exercise and stress management.
Noncompetitive.

Iyengar yoga
Uses props.
Poses held for a minute.
Very slow pace.

Power yoga
Powerful, sweat producing, muscle building.
Intense aerobic workout.

Restorative yoga
Lying on floor.
Depends on blocks, blankets and yoga bolsters.
Passively allowing muscles to relax.

Linda Hoffman

Book III

Vayikra/Leviticus

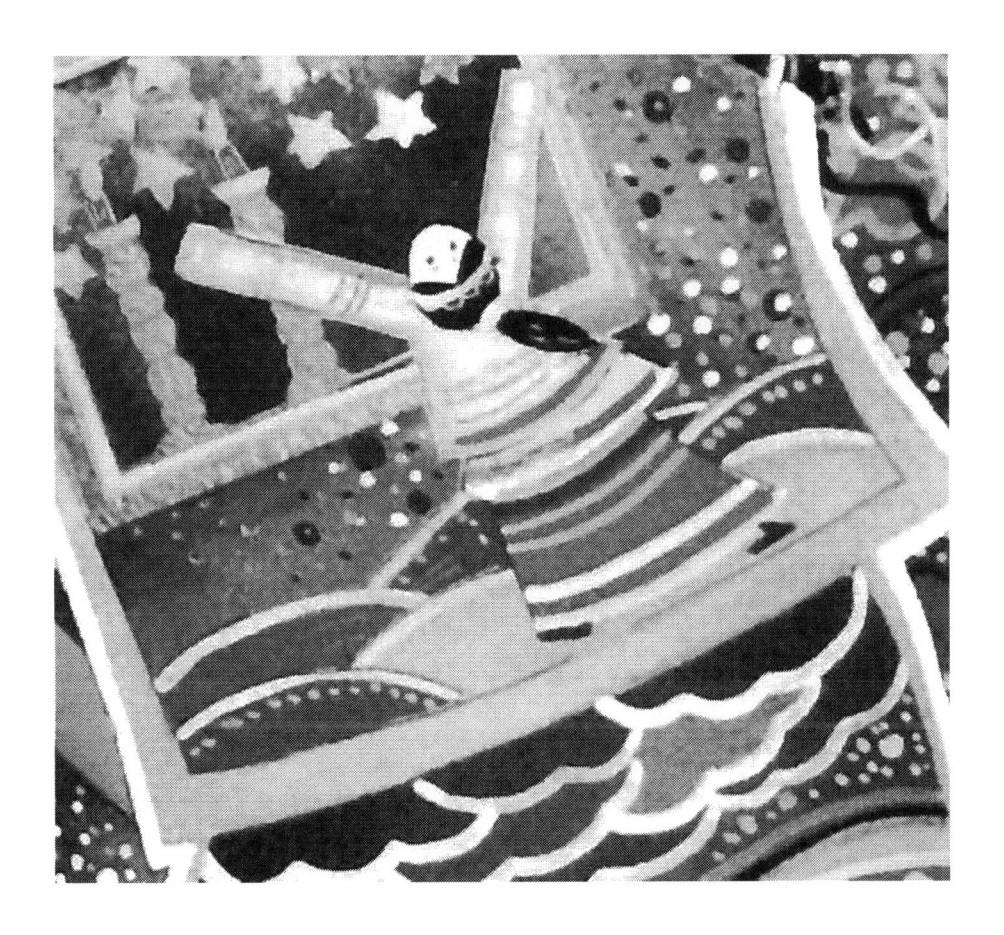

Vayikra (and he called)

Parsha Insight — Offerings

Hashem Calls Moses
The parsha opens with the word vayikra, "and he called." Usually the words "Hashem spoke to Moses and he said" precede the text. The book of Vayikra/Leviticus takes place at the base of Mount Sinai. The people left Egypt, crossed the Yam Suf and arrived at Mount Sinai. What does it means that Hashem says vayikra? This is Hashem lovingly calling Moses. "Moses, come here, listen."

Look in the Chumash and you will see that the parsha starts with the word vayikra. Notice that the final letter, the alef, is smaller than the other letters. Moses, so humble that when he heard Hashem calling him lovingly, wondered about writing a full-size alef. He made a small alef. He did not want to aggrandize himself.

Vayikra is About Sacrifices
Vayikra, the first word of the parsha, tells us about the offerings to Hashem. An offering is an act of humility. An important type of offering is the sin offering. Here, you are making the offering because you did something wrong and you are coming to Hashem in a humble manner and asking for forgiveness. The wrong things that we do are at different levels. A sin is a violation of one of Hashem's mitzvahs, and this violation brings regret. We take a korban, a live creature, as our sacrifice, and slaughter it. The animal stands in our place.

It is hard for us to understand this. We lay hands on the animal, profess our sins, and we know that the animal goes and not us. This mitzvah is from Hashem, but we don't truly comprehend it because of our current sensitivities.

Intent of Offerings
Before Vayikra there were offerings to Hashem. Adam, Cain and Abel made offerings. Cain said to Abel, "Let's make an offering to Hashem." Cain brought flax and Abel brought a sheep. Hashem looked with favor at Abel's offering and not at Cain's. Why did this happen? It wasn't because of the quality of the offering but because of the meaning behind it: the thought, the devotion and the understanding. It is not just the physical act but it is the intent, the meaningfulness, the heartfelt understanding of the situation and our part in it. We come out better than we were before because we learned about our actions and took steps to improve ourselves.

Teshuva
Today if I do something wrong, I don't buy a cow and bring it to my synagogue and kill it on top of the bima (the raised platform in the center of the synagogue). Instead, blessings five, six and seven of the daily Shemoneh Esrei prayer are our prayer for teshuva.

Blessing 5: Repentance
We know we did something wrong, we acknowledge, take ownership.

Blessing 6: Forgiveness
We sinned and ask for a pardon.

Blessing 7: Redemption
We ask to be brought back to where we were before.
Teshuva is repentance, forgiveness and redemption.

Sins of Deed, Speech and Thought
It difficult to figure out all the korbanos, the offerings. You need a chart. For the sins of deed there is the laying of hands. For the sins of speech there is verbal confession. For the sins of thought the animal's heart is burned by fire to consume the thought as it goes up in smoke.

Change Behavior to Change Attitude
The underlying psychology is that behavior affects attitude. When I was in college and majoring in psychology, the behavioral school was in vogue. B. F. Skinner was the leading proponent and showed that by changing behavior, you change attitude. Behavior is a habit. If it is a bad habit, stop doing it, the attitude will change. This Torah portion says the same thing. The behavior exhibited by the ritual will be so disconcerting that our attitude will change.

All sacrifices are not burned up and the ashes thrown away. They are used as a meal. If it is a really terrible sin, we don't want to make a meal out of it. The shared meal with the family at home is sharing a meal with Hashem. Imagine that we brought a korban for a sin, and we saw our wrong, got forgiveness and redemption and then brought the meal home and ate with the family, a meal with God. Korban means to draw near and we draw Hashem near to us and share a meal with Him.

Some mistakes are intentional, we know what we should do but we don't do it. This is the highest level of sin.

The next level is unintentional. We did something, but we didn't think this result would come about. The result is unintentional. Maybe we should have thought a little more about the consequences of our actions. If we do this, then this will occur. We need to be more careful.

The final level is totally accidental, unconscious, we didn't even know it was wrong. We are not sure it was a sin. We still bring an offering because we atone for the carelessness. Did we do a sin? Nah, it is okay. But maybe not. Repent for not watching ourselves enough. We should not hold anyone else to this standard.

Yoga—Pigeon pose

This pigeon is not going to be our sacrifice, but it is going to take some effort.

Start in the downward dog.
Lift your right leg.
Bring right knee to right hand, underneath you.
Lower your body down to floor.
Your left leg is straight back.
Look up with chest out (pigeon with large chest).
Lower to ground with forehead on floor.
Release and the upper part of you rises with chest out.
Twist and look over right shoulder.
Reverse legs and do the other side.

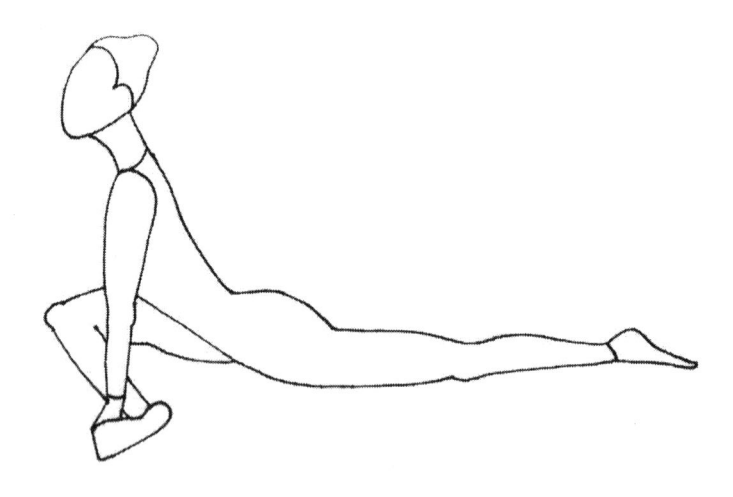

Tzav (Command)

Parsha Insight—Bad thoughts

Thought Offerings
Tzav means command. The word is used as "encouragement" so that the mitzvahs are done with urgency and immediacy. The mitzvahs have continuity and apply to all future generations.

This parsha includes the olah and the elevation offerings which atone for improper thoughts. These offerings are burnt and go up in smoke. What is a thought? We can't touch it, it is like smoke. We have a thought and it can be so fleeting, it is here, it is gone; like smoke, we can't capture it. We are making this offering and sending it up in smoke and we get no benefit from the offering. It is not perfumed to smell better. It is just burnt up into smoke and ash. The ash is important enough that the Kohen Gadol gets dressed in the bigdei kehuna, the priestly garments, to shovel it.

How can our thought be a sin? It's in our head. No one is affected by it. If we don't act on it, nothing happened, right? "Do not stray after your thoughts, and after your eyes..." (Bamidbar/Numbers 15:39). According to Rashi, the eyes see, and the heart desires. If something becomes acceptable in our mind, how easy it is to proceed to acceptable in deed. We protect ourselves and monitor our thoughts. We can stop a negative thought and turn our mind to something more positive. "This is the law of the... (olah offerings)." Since we don't do the olah or thought offerings in these days, studying these laws is as good as if we made the olah offering.

Thanksgiving Offerings
Thanksgiving offerings are called todah offerings and thank Hashem for His blessings. Perhaps the person recovered from an illness. The todah offering includes meat and both leavened and unleavened bread. The unleavened breads stand for miraculous events while the leavened breads stand for natural routines of life. Thanksgiving offerings are enjoyed with family and friends. The person giving the offering tells his story and is praising Hashem in public

Leadership
Moses commanded Aaron to take on the role of the Kohen Gadol. Delegating others to do some of the jobs is leadership. One person can't do everything himself. This is what Yisro told Moses. Moses delegated to Aaron and Aaron's descendants the job of Kohen Gadol. Moses delegated power and responsibility, and that is important. If responsibility is given, the power to make it happen must go with it. Responsibility without the authority is worthless. Moses instructed Aaron on the things he had to do—his responsibilities—and then he let him perform without micromanagement.

Yoga—Deep breathing

We will practice deep breathing to rid us of toxins in our system. Deep, slow breaths rid our system of carbon dioxide and bring lots of fresh oxygen to our brain, our muscles and our blood cells. We can't see these toxins, just as we can't see our sinful thoughts. For bad thoughts, we bring an olah offering, and for bad carbon dioxide toxins we deeply and slowly inhale and exhale.

Toxins are removed by deep exhales from your mouth.
Breathe deeply by inhaling through your nose, to the count of five.
Exhale, through your mouth, to the count of six.
At the top of each inhale, hold for a bit before you exhale.
At the bottom of each exhale, hold for a bit before you inhale.
There is a separation between the inhale and exhale.
Exhaling from the mouth and you feel you are emptying your lungs.
Don't be afraid to make noise while breathing. You will feel a vibration.

Shemini (Eighth)

Parsha Insight — Preparation

Prepare for the Consecration
There were seven days of preparation for Aaron and his four sons before they could be consecrated as Kohanim in the mishkan (tabernacle). For seven days they remained at the entrance of the tent of meeting. During that time, Moses performed the duties of the Kohen Gadol. The consecration of Aaron and his sons took place on the eighth day. Being a Kohen passed from father to son for all future generations. The person who would become the Kohen Gadol was chosen. On the day of the consecration an offering was made and a fire from heaven came and consumed the offering.

Let's back up. Before the seven days of preparation, Moses came to Aaron and told him to come near, come near to me, and let me tell you what your job will be. In last week's parsha, Moses delegated the duties of the Kohen Gadol to Aaron and gave him the responsibility and the authority to do the job. Now he asked Aaron to draw near so that he could tell him about the job and what was expected of him.

Aaron was thinking about his part in the incident of the golden calf and he did not know if he was good enough for this position. He hesitated. He had humility and shame and thought that he could not go forward because he lacked some important qualities. Moses told him not to refrain from doing a mitzvah because of his embarrassment over the golden calf. Moses said that Hashem in his mercy is desiring your service and this is despite anything. All people sin, but your service is still needed. You are still asked to do mitzvahs.

Aaron was told to embolden himself in the service to Hashem and to accept the position of Kohen Gadol. We saw in parsha Tzav that one must do a mitzvah with excitement, with alacrity, and with confidence, and not delay. Aaron was called forward to do this mitzvah with his four sons.

Aaron's Two Oldest Sons
After the consecration, the two oldest sons of Aaron, without discussion with anyone, took it upon themselves to offer a foreign fire to God. This is a fire that is not already in the mishkan and is not a fire requested by Hashem. The fire consumed the offering and the two sons.

Let's equate Aaron and his humility and shame over the golden calf and his two sons' actions. They took it upon themselves to come up with a bigger, better, different way to make an offering to Hashem. The sons were overcome with feelings for Hashem and were functioning out of honorable intent.

We must be very watchful about excessive religiosity. Excessive religious zeal is not acceptable. It is acceptable to follow Hashem's rules. There was no necessity to go over and above. There was no reason for it. While it seems that this was severe punishment, we need to understand that these actions were not those Hashem requested. It was not their job to put themselves in God's place and say in effect, "What you did was pretty good, but watch this."

Laws of Kosher
Right after this incident, the Torah gives us the laws of kosher—the laws pertaining to food. Hashem says, "These are the creatures you may eat." Very specific laws and right after the consecration. We learn that the specific laws of kosher are to be adhered to in the same manner as the specific laws of the consecration. No deviations. We can eat any animal with a double hoof that chews its cud. Even though the pig has double hooves, it does not chew its cud and we cannot eat it. The Torah means exactly what is said.

It is interesting to point out that the giraffe is a kosher animal but we do not eat it. The reason we don't eat the giraffe is because the neck is so long that the rabbis were not sure where on the neck to cut for the kill. Sometimes sticking your neck out is good for you!

We look at the rules of kosher and we try to find reasons for the rules. How come we do not eat shellfish? Are they dirty? We try to find a logical reason. Perhaps we can't eat pork because of trichinosis. We try to comprehend why something is kosher and something else is treif (not kosher).

We are what we eat. To us, this means to eat broccoli and no junk food. Apply this to the laws of kosher and that we eat animals with the appropriate spiritual level. What do we eat—a lamb, a sheep, a goat, a cow; we eat placid and calm animals and put their spirit into ourselves.

Another thought, Hashem says these are the animals you shall eat. He begins with what we may call food. Maybe we can only eat that which we are given permission to call food. We are not entitled to all that is out there. Just because it is available does not mean that it is for us. This removes food from a level of entitlement to a level of permitted.

No Drinking in Shul
You are what you eat, Hashem told Moses. Moses told Aaron that one should not enter the sanctuary after drinking wine. Were the people all drunkards that they had to be told not to drink before entering the sanctuary?

God needs to be experienced in this world without impaired senses, with a clear head. We learn Torah to know and love Hashem. Torah improves our middos, our behavior. We embrace this physical world and make it holy without mind-altering substances. We can't take the secular and make it holy if our mind is impaired by drink or drugs because we can't see things as they are. Our job is to distinguish between the pure and impure, and we can't do that if we are drunk.

Yoga—Get ready for yoga

Before your yoga practice, you need to get ready to do yoga.
You have to get quiet, to calm your body and mind.
Relax. You have no place else to go.
If I have to be someplace in 45 minutes, I can't do a 30-minute yoga practice.
I do not have the proper mindset.

It is the same with Torah learning.
Preparation time is needed to be open and receptive.
Before you begin, take some moments to sit, relax, breathe deeply and clear your mind.
Good to set regular times for Torah study.
Find a comfortable place.
Do not allow anything to interrupt you.
Offer a few words of prayer.
Use deep breathing to renew energy.
(From Azamra.com)

Tazria (she bears seed)
Metzora (infected one)

Parsha Insight — Holy and unholy

No Halfway Measures
In the last parsha we studied what is kosher and what is not kosher. The laws of kosher are strict and there are no halfway measures. Something is either kosher or it is not kosher.

Something is either pure or impure. This is not referring to clean or unclean. The English translation from Hebrew leaves much to be desired as far as getting the correct interpretation of the word impurity. We hear impure, and we immediately think dirty, embarrassing, shameful, even disgusting. Impure means that it is not holy, it is not sanctified.

We eat cows, we do not eat lions. Lions aren't dirty, they are just not kosher. The cows that we eat, the kosher cows, are pure and the lions that we don't eat are impure. The lions aren't bad, they just are not food. What is pure and impure is not a matter for rational determination. God decreed these things and we accept them.

Death is Impure
Death is tameh (impure) and the impurity is transferable. If we touch a dead body, we have death on our person and we then are not pure. There are things that are characteristic of death, that maybe we never thought of that way, that are impure. Each monthly period is a death. Each month, an egg that did not get fertilized is discarded and this flow of blood is impure. A man's nocturnal emission is impure.

To erase the impure and make pure, we go to a mikvah and totally submerge our body in the water. This is a halachic purity, a purity of religious law, and not about clean or unclean. Unfortunately, this causes confusion and, because of lack of understanding, people see dirty in the natural functions of our bodies. This is not in any way to suggest repulsive, unclean, or unsanitary. It represents a death and therefore is impure.

Tzaraas
Tzaraas is a skin infliction that can also be a mar on our clothing or on our house. Today, we go to a dermatologist if we have a spot on our skin. In the years of the Temple, we would go to the Kohen Gadol. Tzaraas is a result of loshon hora, speaking evil. It is the bad use of our mouth. The Kohen Gadol inspects the spot on our skin (on our clothing and our house as well). If the rash on our skin is tzaraas, we are sent out of town, to be by ourselves and consider our actions.

Isolation is a good way to get the sinner to stop gossiping and to think about his actions. He is removed from the town and is alone without anyone to talk to. It is hard to gossip without an audience. He has plenty of time to think.

We need to understand what loshon hora is—how it embarrasses someone. It affects three people: the speaker, the listener and the subject. Three sins committed by talking ugly. Saying something to protect another in a shidduch (matchmaking situation) or a business deal is permitted under certain conditions. Please refer to the book *Guard Your Tongue: A Practical Guide to The Laws of Loshon Hora Based on the Chofetz Chaim* by Rabbi Zelig Pliskin.

The Power of Speech
The power of speech is what distinguishes us from other creatures. You see why it is so important that we guard our speech. I heard this from a rebbetzin in Dallas. There was a fine decanter of wine with a good expensive wine in a beautiful decanter. Unfortunately, there was dirt on the top of the decanter. When the fine wine was poured, the dirt got into the glass. The fine wine was now contaminated by the dirt on the lip of the decanter. The wine can be the best, the decanter and the glasses the finest crystal, but dirt on the mouth of the decanter ruins the whole thing.

Mussar is a Continuum
From impure to pure there is no halfway state. If it is not halachically pure, it is impure. This differs from our personal characteristics. Mussar, our guidelines for living, is our job on earth. We are here to improve ourselves and to use the gifts we receive from Hashem.

We spend our lives enhancing ourselves so that we can be fully actualized. If we are not patient, we strive for patience; but we do not want to be so laid-back that we become a slug. We aim for a midpoint and balance. We want to be able, with discernment, to be patient when needed and proactive when needed. The Rambam said that one way to work on ourselves and come to balance is to force ourselves to the other extreme. This may be very much out of character. Think of it as a way to grow towards the midpoint and to balanced and appropriate responses to situations.

How can we go from no patience to the midpoint? We can add relaxing activities to our day. Take a yoga class, get a massage, take off half a day and read a fun book. Make it happen. Do it, even if, while reading a novel, we find that we are telling ourselves that we must do the hall closet TODAY — NOW.

Yoga—Back bend and forward bend

A back bend is counterbalanced with a forward bend.
Only go as far back and as far forward as you comfortably can.

Raise your arms over your head.
Stand up straight, feet together.
Bend backwards trying to look at the ceiling.

Straighten up and bend forward from the hips.
Move slowly.
Rise up slowly.

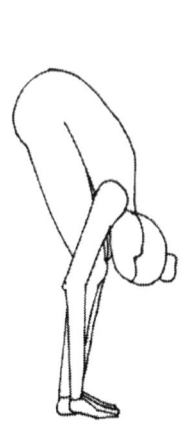

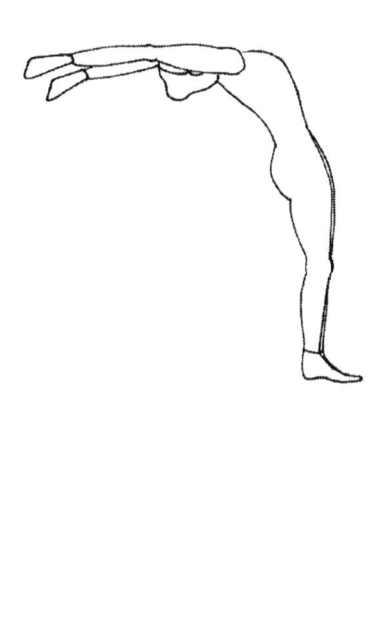

Acharei (after the death)
Kedoshim (Holy ones)

Parsha Insight — Atonement

Atonement
These two parshas are beautiful together. We atone for sins and return to holiness.

Sins atoned for on Yom Kippur are sins against Torah. For these, we ask for forgiveness from Hashem.

Sins against people are acts of an injustice we committed against the person. We first ask the person to forgive us. Then, because we acted against Torah, we ask Hashem to forgive us.

Atonement is awesome because we recognize and acknowledge that we have done wrong. We feel bad and our conscience bothers us. We affirm that we will not do this again.

Atonement is not only a confession of a sin, it is a commitment we make with ourselves, with the other person and with God that we will not do this act again. If we know that we will commit the same sin again, atonement is not appropriate. If we drove on Shabbos and we know that next week we will drive again, atoning for driving on Shabbos is not suitable.

If I apologize to you for loshon hora, gossip, but I can't wait to run to talk about you to someone else, it is not a valid apology. If I knew that as soon as I was out of your sight I would be talking about you again, what kind of apology is that? You would not accept my apology and neither would God.

Atonement is an amazing accountability because we are taking responsibility for our actions. It is not the other person's fault and not God's fault. We have to fix ourselves. We have the obligation to do what is right. This is teshuva, a return to where we were before we committed the offenses. We ask Hashem to put us back to the moral condition we were in before we sinned.

Time of the Temple
When we had the Temple and sacrifices, on Yom Kippur two identical goats were sacrificed to rid us of our sins. By a drawing of lots, so that the decision was determined by God, one goat was sacrificed to the fires. The other goat was sent over a cliff along with all the sins of the population. What symbolism! Goat number one takes our sins and they are turned to smoke. Goat number two bears our sins and takes them over the cliff. The people could grasp this concept because it was tangible.

Many years ago, I attended a class in how to reduce worry. The instructor suggested that the concept be put in tangible form. Like the goats! We were told to visually take all our troubles and put them in a closet and shut the door. This would give us a break from our worries. We still have to solve our problems. We just manage them better.

The two goats are a way for us to breathe deeply and release our guilt. We still have to acknowledge our actions, take steps not to repeat the sin, and improve our behavior.

Can we comprehend the awesomeness of atonement? Only Hashem, in His mercy, could provide us with a way to return to holiness through teshuva. We take a major responsibility for our atonement and our desire to bring holiness back into our lives.

Stay with Torah
Torah tells the Israelites not to follow the practices of Egypt and Canaan. Egypt was where they came from and Canaan was where they were going. Do not act as the people where you had lived acted, and do not do what the people you will encounter do. Stay with Torah. Surrounding the Israelites were people practicing incest, murder and other immoralities. Hashem told the Israelites not to accept their practices and to keep Torah.

Prior to this parsha, when Moses instructed the people on Torah he would tell Aaron, then Aaron's sons, then the rest of the Kohanim and the Levites, then the elders, and finally the people. This section of Torah is so important that everyone was told all at once.

Kedoshim is meant to be understood by all equally, regardless of whether a high priest or an Israelite. The laws apply to everyone equally. Parsha Kedoshim repeats the Ten Commandments.

Kadosh means separate. The Kedoshim are the holy ones and are separate from the people of the other nations. This is the most important parsha of Torah law. It includes the fundamental teachings of Judaism. The most important concept of Judaism is to "love your neighbor as yourself." The parsha Kedoshim and "love your neighbor as yourself" is in the middle of the Torah. This is central to Torah and is essential to being a person, a mensch.

What does "love your neighbor as yourself" mean? How can we possibly love our neighbor as ourselves? It means do no harm. Do not put a stumbling block in another's way. Do not cause harm. Do what we can to ward off a problem. Do what is within our power to protect another.

Create a Plan for Teshuva

The goal of Torah is to make the secular holy. Our body is secular and our deeds, words and thoughts make it holy. We have to look at things ethically and morally. If we change our behavior and our speech, our thoughts change. Teshuva provides us with a system to examine and enhance our lives. This is Torah. By changing our actions, we see the world differently.

How do we formally correct what is wrong? Do we talk about it? Do we create actions to fix? How can we return to where we were before? We need teshuva to set aside the negative so we can move on. Thoughts are fleeting like smoke. We need to create a plan.

Make a Plan for Teshuva
Set a goal.
Create a procedure for change.
Evaluate progress periodically.
Plan a reward for success.

Yoga—Concentration

When you do yoga, are you emptying your mind of everything? Do you have a blank mind? No, that is not yoga, that's a coma!

Yoga does not empty your mind, it makes you more mindful. As we go through the poses, we pay attention to our body and our breath. We are focusing intently. It's amazing but when you are thinking about your breath, no other thoughts are in your mind. That is why it is usually recommended that a pose be held for five complete breaths. First you get into the pose, concentrating on your body's position, and then you remain in the position and focus on your breath. It will take some practice to build your ability to stay with the pose for this length of time.

When we study Torah we need the same intensity—100% mindful of what we are reading. Prayer requires 100% focus. Sometimes we pray by rote. We are not listening to our own words.

We get up in the morning. Say Modei Ani. Wash our hands. Pour a glass of orange juice. Say the blessing h'aretz (blessing for food growing on trees) and then wonder—Did I wash my hands? Why? Because we were not mindful, we operated on rote. If we were mindful and conscious of washing the hands, thinking of washing away the night, the 1/60 of death of sleep, thankful that we woke this morning, grateful to Hashem, mindful of what we are doing, then we would remember that we washed our hands. The experience becomes more powerful and meaningful.

Yoga teaches concentration. Yoga teaches you to focus on one thing and only one thing at a time. Yoga keeps the "monkey brain" and all its distractions away. The monkey brain is all that chatter that goes on in our minds. It is not accomplishing anything because usually it is just a broken record of the same thought over and over again. When my monkey brain goes into automatic pilot, I take a pencil and paper (sometimes make a note on my iPhone if I remember to use it) and write out that repetitious thought. Once I make it tangible, it leaves my mind. I have it on my list of things to do. I will get to it. It just does not need to mess with my concentration right now.

A very visual student in class saw her yoga practice as a funnel of what is happening around her. She narrows the field and focuses on one thing. This is like a laser beam pointing her in the proper direction and leading her on. Today, do your normal yoga practice, but focus on your mindfulness.

Emor (say)

Parsha Insight—Character improvement

The duties and laws of the Kohanim are in this parsha. The Kohen has a responsibility to sustain higher standards of holy behavior and purity than the rest of the nation. Aaron was the first Kohen and all his descendants are Kohanim. It passes from father to sons. The Kohanim cannot touch a dead body. Kohanim cannot marry a harlot or a divorcee. I have always found it unfortunate that both words are used in the same posik (verse).

The Kohanim Have to Be Pure
To perform the Temple service, Torah says that the Kohen may not have any blemish or deformity. He must be perfect. A blemish may be lameness, sickness, scarring, etc.

What about today? Today, a Kohen may do the first aliyah (first blessing of Torah reading) regardless of whether or not he has any blemishes, but he cannot do the priestly blessings. The priestly blessings are said on Yom Tovim (holy days). All the Kohanim walk out of the room for the ritual washing and those with a blemish do not return until the blessings are done. This is done so that no one is aware if anyone is missing.

Excluding people with blemishes does not sound good to us with our current perception of political correctness and with the Americans with Disabilities Act. Hashem is wise in understanding us and knows that, although we have good intentions, we stare at the disabled and are distracted by differences. Torah is making sure we focus on the blessings and not on the Kohen's deformity or blemish.

Festivals Established
In this parsha, the festivals of Passover, Rosh Hashanah, Sukkos, Shemini Atzeres, Shavuos and Yom Kippur are established and described. Shabbos is included with these festivals. Shabbos is so special that even though it occurs every week, it deserves mention along with the festivals.

The festival of Yom Kippur is the Day of Atonement. There are five afflictions of Yom Kippur and each is paired with a sin for which we atone.

No food: pairs with the sin of food, any non-kosher food we may have had during the year.
No drink: pairs with the sin of any inappropriate drink we may have had during the year. Maybe drinking to excess, or a dairy drink with or following a meat meal.

No leather shoes: pairs with running to do a sin.

No washing or anointing: pairs with forbidden pleasures.

No marital relations: pairs with the sin of inappropriate sexual activity during the year.

Atonement and teshuva (usually translated as repentance) return us to a clean slate. We return to the individual we were before the sin. You can't atone for a sin that you intend to repeat. To do so is said to be like going to a mikvah (a ritual bath used to purify us) with a dead animal in our hands. We can't return clean if we don't recognize and agree not to repeat a sin.

Passover

Passover is the festival to commemorate our leaving Egypt and our nation being created.

When the Jews left Egypt, they were at the forty-ninth level of impurity. This means that they had adopted just about all the Egyptian ways. One more level and they would have been completely lost.

We count the Omer for fifty days from the second night of Passover till Shavuos. You count forward and the fiftieth day is Shavuos, when we got the Torah. Counting the Omer to fifty reminds us that we were saved and came to Torah.

In Pirkei Avos 6.6 are listed the forty-eight steps to character improvement. Torah values are acquired with these forty-eight attributes.

The counting and the Pirkei Avos usually go together even though the Omer just counts. Our job is to improve ourselves and our middos, our personal qualities. We improve ourselves and become the best "me" that we can be.

"Study, listening, verbalizing, comprehension of the heart, awe, fear, humility, joy, purity, serving the sages, companionship with one's contemporaries, debating with one's students, tranquility, study of the scriptures, study of the Mishnah, minimizing engagement in business, minimizing socialization, minimizing pleasure, minimizing sleep, minimizing talk, minimizing gaiety, slowness to anger, good heartedness, faith in the sages, acceptance of suffering, knowing one's place, satisfaction with one's lot, qualifying one's words, not taking credit for oneself, likableness, love of G-d, love of humanity, love of charity, love of justice, love of rebuke, fleeing from honor, lack of arrogance in learning, reluctance to hand down rulings, participating in the burden of one's fellow, judging him to the side of merit, correcting him, bringing him to a peaceful resolution [of his disputes], deliberation in study, asking and answering, listening and illuminating, learning in order to teach, learning in order to observe, wising one's teacher, exactness in conveying a teaching, and saying something in the name of its speaker." (Pirkei Avos)

A wonderful essay by Rabbi Noah Weinberg from Aish.com, "Change Your Life with the Forty Eight Ways," is recommended for additional reading about our middos.

Yoga—Warrior success pose

Warrior success pose — arms up
A pose of balance and strength to remember our success with the forty-eight ways of self-improvement in Pirkei Avos.

Stand with legs together.
Step right leg forward.
Right foot flat on ground.
Left foot with heel lifted and toe on ground.
Bend your right leg at the knee.
Arms up.
There will be a curve to your spine as you look up.
Come out of pose slowly and bring feet together.
Now do the other side.
Left leg stepping forward.
Left foot flat on ground.
Right foot with heel lifted and toe on ground.
Bend your left leg at the knee.
Arms up.
There will be a curve to your spine as you look up.
Come out of pose slowly and bring feet together.

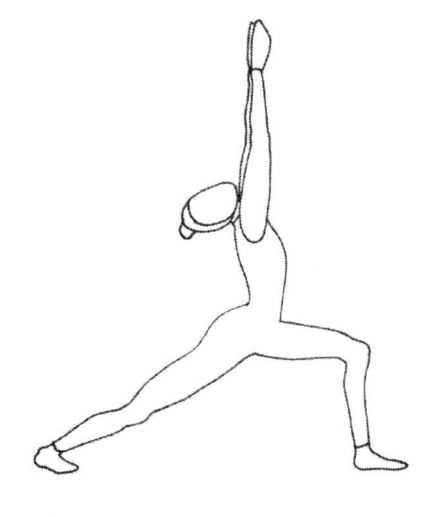

Behar (on the Mount)
Bechukotal (in My Statutes)

Parsha Insight — No coincidence

Book of Vayikra Begins and Ends With Korbanos
In the beginning of Vayikra, the korban (offering) described is a sin offering. At the end of Vayikra, the korban is a tithe offering. Korbanos, offerings, were given as part of teshuva, returning to a state of purity from sin. We have obligations to do teshuva for our sins and we have an obligation to the Jewish Nation to contribute our fair share to charity. Giving charity is often part of the teshuva process. With a korban offering we are drawing near to God and to community.

Freedom from Slavery
In the last parsha, Emor, we studied the counting of the Omer and the mussar (behavioral) steps in Pirkei Avos. This is our personal journey in Torah understanding, self-improvement and internal freedom. The turmoil of negative impulses impacts our choices and we are in personal oppression. Character trait improvement helps us develop freedom from emotional slavery.

If I am jealous of others, I see events with a jaundiced eye. I see other people getting rewards and wonder, where are my good tidings? How come they have them and I don't? I am a slave to my jealousy and will not be free until I change my behavior. Once I see the good things in my life, value them and have gratitude for what Hashem gave me, I will not be jealous of someone else's life. I become emotionally free. I also become free to rejoice in their successes.

In Behar we learn that the fiftieth year, the Yovel, is a count to liberty. Indentured servants are freed. The Yovel year is a physical freedom from slavery. In putting together this writing, I discovered that the Liberty Bell in Philadelphia says, "Proclaim Liberty throughout all the Land unto all the Inhabitants thereof." That comes from Behar 25:10, referring to the Yovel year and the freedom for all Jewish slaves.

No Coincidences
In Bechukotal we are given a rebuke. If we don't follow Hashem's ways, if we are casual in our observance, Hashem will be casual with us. If we think that incidents happen haphazardly or are a coincidence, Hashem will withdraw and leave us to our own devices. Hashem created the universe and continues to create. Everything that happens comes from God.

Look back over the past several years and the events in your own life. See how the pieces have come together. Doesn't it seem as though a master conductor choreographed everything? Ask yourself, if you hadn't (for example) moved to a new city, would you have had certain experiences? What did you learn from those events? Have you grown? Could it all have been by chance? Would you want a life determined by the throw of the dice?

Yoga–Discipline

To get the most benefit from our yoga practice, we need to apply our personal discipline and be consistent in our exercise program. Being casual doesn't work, not in yoga and not in our observances.

It is good to do yoga at a bare minimum two times a week.
Find a practice that incorporates total body movement.
Your goal is to improve your flexibility and mobility.
If you work regularly on your yoga, you will see improvement in your posture, your outlook, your attention span, and you will be able to move about more freely.

I wish I could tell you that you will lose weight, but yoga is not an exercise for weight reduction.
For that, add a short daily walk to your practice and reduce food intake.
Eat more vegetables and fruit and don't take up crash diets.
Steady and consistent!

Book IV

Bamidbar/Numbers

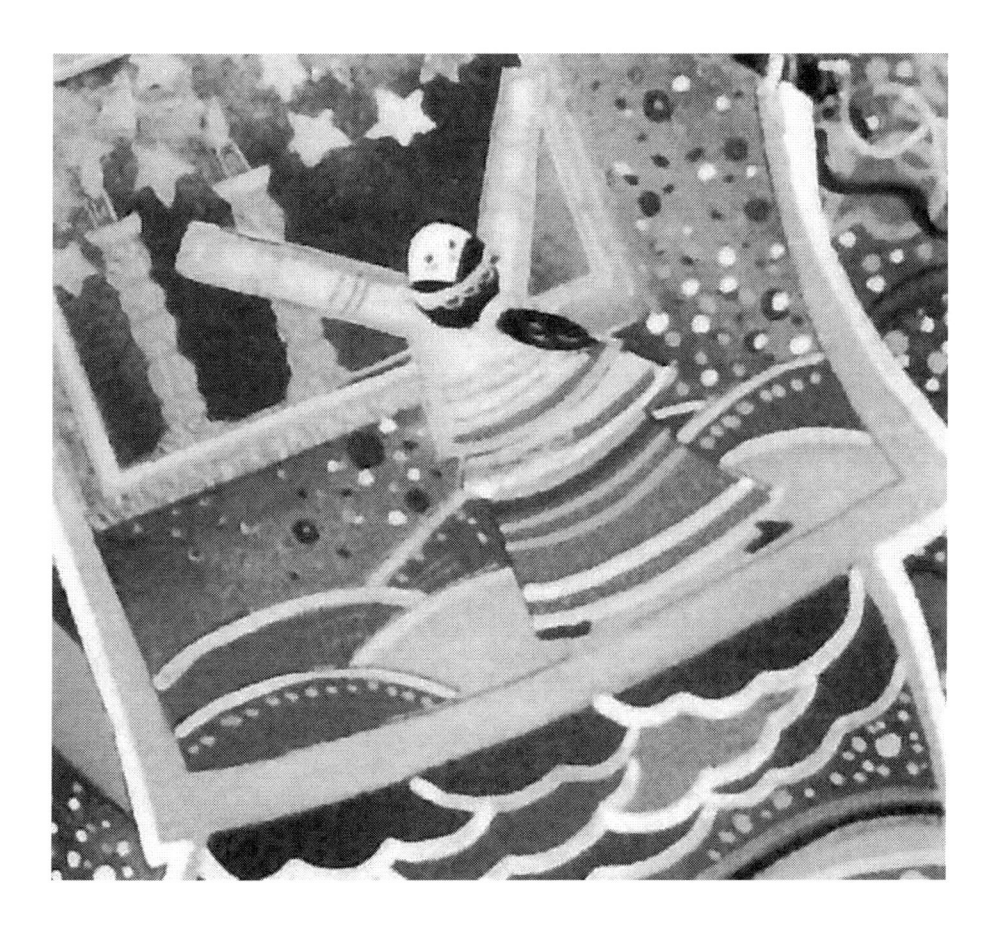

Bamidbar (in the desert)

Parsha Insight — Know your place

Positions in camp and traveling
In this parsha we take a census that differs from all other censuses. A personal count was made by Aaron and Moses just before the Jewish Nation left Mount Sinai. Each able-bodied male over twenty years of age came before them and was counted. The count was made with Hashem resting His presence among them. The phrase "Take a Census" also means an elevation of the heads. This census lifted up the heads so that each man knew his worth and his part in the Jewish Nation.

Bamidbar (in the desert) represents a formative period for each individual Jew as he connected with his immediate group, the larger family, the community and to the nation as a whole. We see by the personal count that each person was important. Each man lifted up his head in pride both as an individual and as belonging to the Jewish Nation.

The words commanding the taking of the census were that Moses and Aaron should count every able-bodied male over the age of twenty, everyone who goes out to the legion (the army). This census was not just for the pride of the individual in the Jewish Nation. It was also to count the number of persons able to protect and defend the people as they left Mount Sinai. I'm sure you noticed that women and children and the aged were not included in this census. Talmud says that no men over sixty were counted in this census.

Know Your Place
In the desert, the camps were arranged by families. Three tribes formed a cluster. The Tabernacle was in the center with the Levites. There was a cluster on each side of the Tabernacle: the North, South, East and West. As they camped, so they walked in the wilderness. Walking and camping with your family, your tribe, in your cluster, and as part of the whole had to be very comforting. You feel secure in your position.

The arrangement of the tribes surrounding the mishkan (tabernacle) was the same as the arrangement of Yaakov's twelve sons when they carried his coffin. The placement was already established; no one would be questioning their place because they already knew it. When you know your place, you accept it with calmness.

I remember our family gathering around the table for dinner. My father always sat in the same place and each of us in the family had our special seat. I don't remember who or what situation assigned the seat, but I knew MY seat and that's the place where I wanted to sit. The only time there was ever a problem was when we had guests and seating was changed to accommodate additional people. There was some grumbling, but as long as each of us was in a position that resembled the prior position, it was acceptable.

Count the Levites
Moses was told by God to count the Levites, including the infants. Moses did not know how he would count the infants without invading on the privacy of the tents. God said, you do your task and I will do mine. We supply our effort and God will do His job.

See the Outcome
This is a good lesson for all of us. We each have to find the proper balance of hishtadlus (our effort) and bitachon (our trust). At what point do we put in more effort and at what point do we trust that Hashem will make sure that the best thing for us will occur? I pray with my own words and ask God to show me the correct action, to give me the wisdom to see the proper action.

The Talmud in Tractate Tamid says, "Who is wise? He who sees the likely outcome of events." Seeing the outcome gives you an inkling into how much effort you need to exert to make something happen. Maybe what you are seeking is not so good for you. Maybe it is just perfect. Either way, you are getting insight into the amount of effort required.

Yoga—Body placement, triangle pose

In this pose we are paying attention to individual parts of our bodies and concentrating on the positioning of our legs, arms, and hips. The total pose is a bending and stretching exercise. We shall flow from standing through the triangle formation. This is the process from single body part, to combination of body sections, to total body movement.

As we saw in the parsha, the individual person has to be recognized first, then the connection to family, to community, and to nation.

Stand with legs mat-width apart.
Hold arms wide out at shoulder height.
Get good balance and keep legs straight.
Pivot on your left heel so the left foot is sideways.
Right foot is forward.
Swing hip to the right, reach left arm as far to the left.
Bend down to the left foot, left arm down, right arm up, look at right arm.
Change sides.

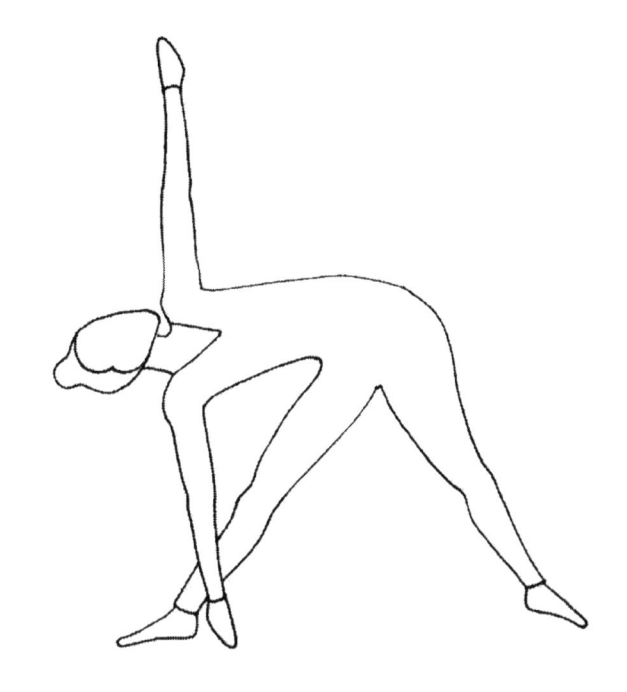

Nasso (elevate)

Parsha Insight—Special each time

Laws of Society
This is the longest parsha in Torah. It has many different topics and laws. The common thread that binds the various laws of Nasso is living peacefully in a society. We are building a nation, and in the previous parsha we saw how we individually functioned within family, community and country. Now we're focusing on social functioning.

Peaceful families trust each other. If a man wrongfully thinks his wife is deceiving him, she drinks a potion with God's name in it. Her innocence is proven by God's name being erased and nothing happens to the wife. Hashem is so concerned with shalom bayis, peace in the home, that he would rather have his name erased than have a husband doubt his wife.

A peaceful society is needed when there is close proximity of people living and working together. Stealing, murder, loshon hora (evil speech) or adultery would cause contention and could pit families and tribes against each other.

No Jealousies
Each of the tribes brought offerings on different days. Amazingly, all of the offerings were the same. There was no envy, no jealousy, and no one was trying to outdo the other. While the offerings were exactly the same, the reasons behind the offerings had different meaning to each of the tribes. Each offering was seen by Hashem as special. It did not make any difference that it was the same as the previous one because each tribe was unique.

You and I both bring our Torah teacher a shiny, red, delicious apple. I chose an apple because I want her to have good health. You chose the apple because you knew she doesn't take the time for a full lunch and you thought she might like a snack.

Suppose we have several children and they each decided to give us a hairpin for our birthday. Each child's gift is special and each child is loved. The gift from each child is lovingly accepted because it is coming from a beloved child. Somehow, we will find a way to put all the hairpins in our hair.

Same Prayer is Special Each Time
This also applies to us and our prayers. We repeat the same prayer each day. We say the same words each day. Shabbos prayers differ. Nevertheless, each prayer is special and we say it with the fervor of new words on our tongue. Sometimes we seem to understand a particular section in our prayers better one day than on other days. We emphasize those parts of the prayer more fully. Maybe our budget is a little tight and we need just a few more sales to make it through the month. The section of the Shemoneh Esrei prayer on parnassah, livelihood, is more to the point today.

Yoga—Each day different

I do the same yoga practice every day. I try to do yoga five times a week. I have my yoga routine on my iPad as a twenty-five-minute audio. I start the same, proceed just as I did the day before, I put the same attention into the positions as the day before. I know that tomorrow I will give my yoga practice the same care.

I recognize that some days I have more energy and my yoga reflects this added energy. Other days, I'm a bit lethargic and the twenty-five minutes seem to take an hour.

I know that my yoga time is special and desired. It is in my best interest to keep the practice fresh each time. Even after many years, I still get a new insight into a pose. For example, recently, while doing the mountain pose, the leader on the audio said lift your knees. Lift your knees! How do you lift your knees while standing tall? Guess what? I got it! It suddenly had meaning and my mountain pose got straighter and my knees seemed to be lifting.

You are reading this and maybe something you do each day comes to mind. Next time, give it a bit of conscious thought. You may surprise yourself and have a new insight.

Beha'alosecha (in your making go up)

Parsha Insight — Blow your own horn

Kindle the Lamps
When you light the menorah, the candelabra, be mindful. Kindling the lamps, Moses very specifically tells Aaron, requires that you take care while lighting. Menorah refers to Torah and the light of Torah refers to our Torah learning. Take care in teaching Torah. Don't do it haphazardly.

When we light Shabbos candles, we strike the match and bring it to the candle wick. We hold the match to the wick until it lights up. We wait until the candle has a separate and distinct flame from the match. Aaron was told to take similar care in lighting the menorah in the mishkan, the tabernacle.

Move 'Em Out!
All of the action in this parsha is happening about a year after leaving Egypt. The people are at the foot of Mount Sinai. They traveled according to the word of God. Travel was not determined by Moses. He didn't just think it was time to move and say, "Move 'em out." Travel was determined by Hashem using the Clouds of Glory. When the clouds were over the encampment, the people stayed put. When the clouds lifted, the people moved. They did not move on their own. They moved according to Hashem's will.

Clouds of Glory

Let's consider this metaphor in our life. When we are depressed, it is hard for us to move. We can't change anything. We feel as though we have no power. The dark clouds are upon us. We are not looking for something new. We are not trying anything out. The clouds are keeping us down. When the clouds were over the Jews they stayed put, they didn't move. Just like us. When the clouds lift, we open up. We feel expanded, we get new ideas, we will try something out, and we will have an adventure. The Clouds of Glory parallel this.

What is raising and lowering our clouds? Is this the hand of God? Is that what tells us to go forward or not?

We have heard the expression "red flag." It is the alert that we get from what is around us. We need to heed these messages because they are telling us when to proceed and when not. It is easy to overlook these signs because they don't seem firm enough. We can find excuses. Pay attention to your "Clouds of Glory." Paying attention to red flags is an active thing. It means getting more information and evaluating what we find out. So when the red flags are waving, let's investigate further and see if we can pinpoint what got our attention.

Laws of Shabbos

The laws of Shabbos come from the thirty-nine major task categories of the building of the mishkan. The activities which are prohibited on Shabbos are the actions of building the mishkan. An interesting point is the law of dismantling and rebuilding. The law is that we cannot dismantle on Shabbos to rebuild on the same site. We can dismantle on Shabbos to rebuild in a different location. This comes from the dismantling of the camps and the rebuilding of the camps. We would say that the camps were dismantled here and rebuilt there. But since in the desert the camps were dismantled and rebuilt under Hashem's will, under the Clouds of Glory, this occurred in the same places. Therefore, these acts are forbidden on Shabbos.

Think of mom carrying a baby. Mom is going to the store, walking on the street, stopping at a neighbor's house—different places. But where is the baby—on Mom's hip. The same place. When I am on a ship, the ship is moving, but I'm in the same place. A fly in my car is in the same place, even though I drove fifty miles.

Make a Trumpet for Yourself
This command is not like making the menorah or the shulchan (table) for the Temple, items that are passed down for generations. You make a trumpet for yourself. Our vernacular is "Blow your own horn." A trumpet sound is the shofar. It is a piercing, soul-wrenching sound. It is a sound that you remember, a sound that becomes embedded in you. The shofar sound keys into the soul and the spirit. It is a personal call to Hashem. We each make our own trumpet. I hear my trumpet with my interpretation. That trumpet is only for me. I must blow my own horn. I learn what the sages teach; then I reflect upon my feelings and understandings of Hashem and not those of anyone else.

Where's the Meat?
This saying comes from a TV commercial some years ago for a fast food hamburger. It's practically a quote from our parsha.

The Jews complained to Moses that they wanted meat. Meat is a symbol of paganism, which is different from idol worship. Idol worship is creating a thing and crediting it with the powers of a god. One meaning of paganism or barbarianism is wanting all the things outside of me and making them mine. It is uncontrolled desire for things outside of myself. I concentrate too much on things and not on my self-development or my soul-development. It is desire gone berserk. It could be overeating, gambling, sex or money. It is a craving without restraints.

Why were the people focusing on meat? They were eating manna that fell from heaven and became any taste and any texture that the people wanted. They could have conjured up meat. Why demand meat? What is this representing?

It symbolizes uncontrolled desires, urgency for things and wanton indulgence. This bothered Moses more than the golden calf. You would think that building a golden calf a short time after hearing Hashem at Mount Sinai would be the worst possible action. Unrestrained behavior is worse. It is all about things and getting what you want when you want it. Torah learning teaches us the mastery over our desires and impulses. By knowing, understanding and controlling our desires, we make the physical holy.

Yoga—Eagle

When in the middle of a yoga pose, stay focused and don't think about the shopping list or fidgeting and readjusting our clothing. We practice mastery over the physical for the benefit of the mind. We are growing and learning in our yoga practice and in our Torah study.

Soar like an eagle. Master the physical. The eagle pose is standing on one leg and wrapping the other leg around the standing leg; the arms are also crossed with palms together and lowered to chest.

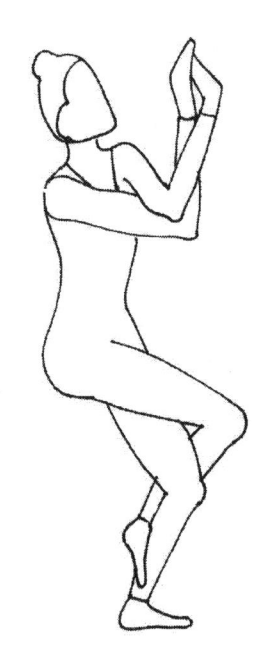

Eagle
In a standing position, bend your knees.
Put the right leg over the left knee, as if you are crossing your legs.
Your right foot is resting on the left calf.
You can hold your arms straight out.
A more challenging arm position is crossing your arms, left over right, try to touch palms.
Lower your crossed arms to the chest.
Bend slightly from the knees.
Your back will arch a little.
Now do the other leg.

Parsha and Yoga

Shelach (send for yourself)

Parsha Insight — As you see yourself

Incident of the Spies
Hashem spoke to Moses and said, "Send forth men if you please and let them spy out Canaan, one from each tribe and each one a leader."

Twelve men went to check out the land the people were going to enter. The spy mission was not a negative event. They were going into a new land and Hashem said that if they wished they could have an advance team explore. Moses asked them to find out answers to very specific questions.

Scoping out something ahead of time is sometimes very beneficial. If I have to be someplace unfamiliar and it is very important that I be on time, I might do a dry run the day before so that I know the lay of the land. Is traffic heavy? Can I make a right turn over here? Answers to these kinds of questions will make my drive the next day easier.

Moses did not ask the spies for their interpretation. Their mission was to look and report the facts about the land, the population, if the cities are walled, and about the weather. Ten of the spies came back with a negative report. The other two spies, Joshua and Calev, did not give a negative report.

Hashem did not need the answers as to the merits of the land. Who needed the answers? The people needed the answers. Moses could have said, "Hashem said the land is good; let's go." It would be much more convincing to have the leaders of the tribes come back and tell the people what Hashem already knew. The land was good. It was a land of milk and honey. The trees had fruit.

Report of the Ten
First
They responded to the intelligence gathering questions by saying that it was indeed a land of milk and honey.

Then, but
BUT: and we know what "but" does. But says forget about everything I said before; this is what I'm saying now. BUT, the people are giants. They are more powerful than us, implying that they are more powerful than God. This section negated the previous answers to specific questions and moved things out of proportion.

Finally
We were like grasshoppers. What does that mean? We are nothings. We are like the grasshopper that crawls on the ground. What right do we have to go there? Why did the spies have no faith in themselves? Why did they have no faith in Hashem?

Possible Reasons for Report
It had been so very easy traveling under Hashem's grace.
Once they got to Israel they would have to take care of themselves.
They would no longer be protected by the Clouds of Glory.
Everything was changing and everything was going to be different.
People fear something different. It is scary.
Different circumstances require change and adaptation.
People get more attention with a negative report than a positive report.

As they related their report, a worsening picture of what they encountered in Canaan developed.

Joshua and Calev
Calev's nature was to wait for the proper opportunity before speaking. Joshua was the type of man to put up resistance to others, in this case the other ten. Moses prayed for Joshua because he knew that Joshua needed prayers for patience.

Joshua and Calev portray two different ways that we deal with adversity. Some of us stick our elbows out, scream and yell, resisting any way we can. Others are more patient and quietly wait for the right time to have their say. When they speak, they say it one time with conviction and without ranting and raving. Moses prayed for Joshua because he knew that Joshua's nature was more explosive and would put up resistance. Moses did not want the differing reports to cause a major fight among the people.

What is the Sin of the Spies?
The sin is that they were sent out on a specific mission and returned with a report that was out of proportion. They agitated the people, and made them hysterical. The people were crying for naught. Hashem said that if you are crying over this, I'll give you something to really cry about. The 9th of Av became the day of crying.

The sin of loshon hora—harmful speech—was also committed by the spies because they told a mistruth. They ran to do harm and they got the people all upset. Loshon hora harms the people who speak, those who listen, and those spoken about, in this case the land.

Hashem's understanding of the people's readiness for living freely in Israel changed. Hashem saw that the people could not get from bondage to freedom. We needed to travel for a total of forty years so that the people of slavery would die out. The children of these people would enter Israel without the memory of Egypt and bondage.

Yom Kippur and Tisha B'Av
Yom Kippur is about teshuva (repentance) and return to holiness. On Yom Kippur we recognize our sins, the wrongs we have done and the lapses we had. We acknowledge what was, we know we are not going to do it again and we ask for forgiveness.

If you do something and you know that you are going to do it again, it is not a proper teshuva. If you drive on Shabbos and you know that you will drive again on the next Shabbos, it is not teshuva to ask for forgiveness on Yom Kippur. Better to accept, I drive on Shabbos so that I can go to shul. Not good, but better, since it is not a pretense of doing teshuva for something that you know you are not going to change.

Tisha B'Av is not about teshuva. It is about mourning the loss of personal vision. The biggest sin of the spies is that they lost faith in themselves. They had a failure to strive.

How We See Ourselves
Think about yourself and when you are feeling good about yourself. You feel like you have the ability to manage life. You can go through things and find the right channels. You won't know all the answers, nevertheless, you feel confident that with Hashem's help, you will find the way.

When we are down, we let the negative feelings permeate our entire understanding of life. We don't even have the confidence to make dinner. Suddenly everything looks bad. Everybody else is wonderful and I'm a nothing. This is a terrible disservice to ourselves.

Hashem made us and He did a good job. Hashem's judgment of us is based on our faith in ourselves. We have to be mindful of how we see ourselves because that is how God sees us. It is also how others see us.

When we are down on ourselves, people see us as a victim and they take advantage of us. When we feel powerful and strong, those people who are looking for victims do not come to us because we won't be an easy candidate for them. They are looking for victims and we are showing them—"Not me, buddy; go someplace else."

Yoga—Strongest warrior

Great for balance and strength.
Stand tall with arms raised up.
Bend forward at the hips.
Your arms are now straight out and forward.
Get your balance.
Raise the right leg.
Hold and breathe.
Bring right leg down.
Raise up to standing tall with arms up.
Bend forward at the hips.
Your arms are straight out and forward.
Regain your balance.
Raise the left leg.
Hold and breathe.
Bring left leg down.
Raise up to standing tall with arms up.
Lower arms.

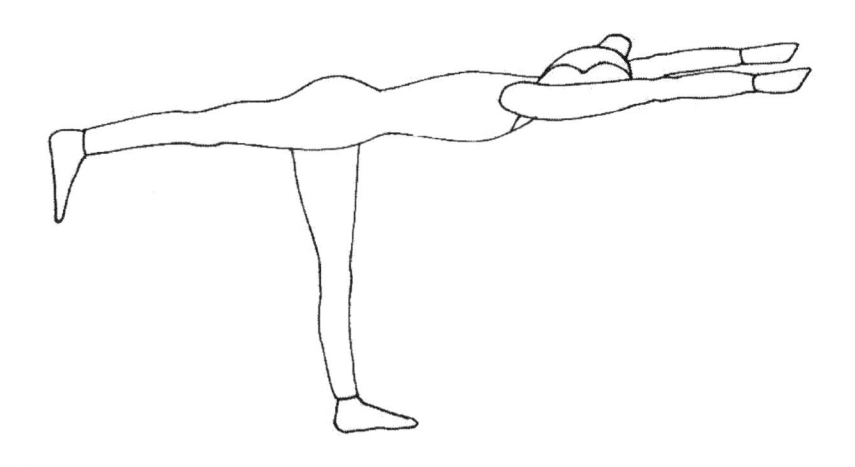

Linda Hoffman

Korach (bald)

Parsha Insight — Not everyone a leader

Questioning
The parsha opens with "Korach...son of a Levi, separated himself..." This refers to Korach seeking discord. Note that the name Korach means bald. All the Levites had shaved heads.

Korach assembled a cohort of two hundred and fifty, all men from leadership positions, to rebel against Moses and Aaron. They asked clever questions about tzitsis (specially tied fringes such as those on prayer shawls) and mezuzah. These were questions that indicated knowledge of Torah rules, but questioned the logic of the mitzvah. They asked if an all-blue, four-cornered garment still requires a blue thread on the tzitsis, or if a house full of seforim, holy books, still requires a mezuzah on the doors. An example of a similar type of question would be me asking about saying the Modeh Ani prayer, which is said upon arising in the morning, if I wake at three in the morning to go to the bathroom.

These questions are saying, "I know what Hashem said. I want to use my common sense. Is this mitzvah logical?" It is not an honest question. It is more about proving that you know better than Hashem. Questioning in this manner is ridiculing the mitzvahs rather than trying to understand and learn Torah.

Not a Dispute for the Sake of Heaven
The dispute of Korach against the authority of Moses and Aaron was not a dispute for the sake of heaven. When Hillel and Shammai (Torah sages) argued about a Torah mitzvah or a Torah learning, they argued so they could better understand Hashem's ways. It was not a personal argument or an argument for personal gain. It was an argument for greater comprehension of God's words.

Korach rebelled because he did not accept that Hashem asked Moses to choose Aaron for the position of Kohen Gadol. He did not accept that Aaron and his sons would be Kohanim. Each of the two hundred and fifty men who joined Korach had his own agenda. We see that the uprising of Korach's was not for the sake of heaven. It was for the sake of personal gain. Each of the men had his individual desires and each caused machlokes (trouble, discord) because he wanted to rule instead of Moses and Aaron. Korach and several of his men were first sons, and they wanted to return power to the first sons.

Fell on His Face
"Moses heard and fell on his face." Falling on one's face is ominous. It is like a loud, ringing bell, a sign to get your attention. It also is a metaphor for embarrassment or disgust for the situation. This was the fourth distressing event since the giving of the Ten Commandments and Torah. We had the golden calf, the complaints requesting meat, the sin of the spies and now the Korach rebellion. After three negative occurrences, we see habitual behavior. Were sin and complaints so much a part of the people's life? Could Moses possibly expect Hashem to excuse the Jewish people yet again?

Strong Message
Korach and his men were swallowed up by the earth. Moses felt that something additional was necessary to show that Hashem's laws prevail. The people needed to see something positive and creative rather than only the destruction of Korach and his followers. Moses asked each of the twelve tribes to take a staff and put its leader's name on it. The staff of the Levites had Aaron's name on it. The staves were put in the ground and Moses said that the one that bloomed was the staff of the leader. The next day Aaron's staff bloomed and the others did not. Aaron's staff was placed in the mishkan for all to see.

Yoga—Pyramid

A pyramid is wide on the bottom and very narrow at the top. Not everyone can get to the top. Korach confused our all being holy with our all being equal. He overlooked that we all do not deserve or belong at the top. We are not all equal. We each have different qualities and abilities and different jobs to do in this life. Everybody can't rule.

Feet apart.
Arms out.
Right leg forward.
Bring arms down and back.
Bend from the hips and lean over the right leg.
Come to center and then do the other side.

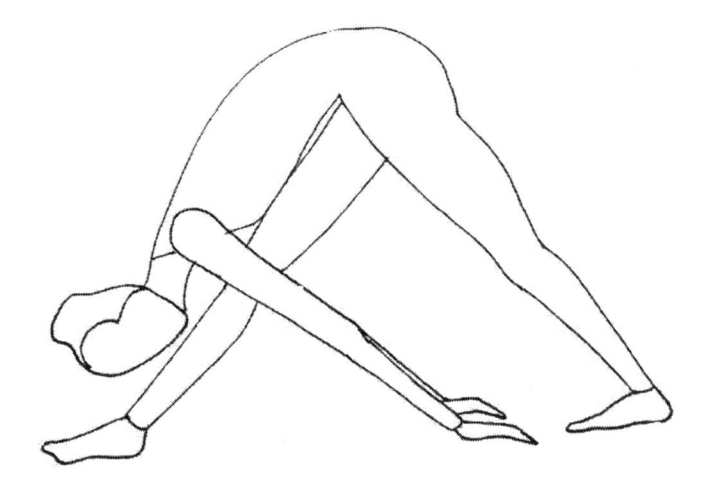

Chukas (ordinance of)

Parsha Insight—Why should I?

Chukas are mitzvah that do not seem logical. The parsha begins with the chok of the red cow. The ashes of the red cow make impure the pure, and pure the impure. What does this mean? Let's come back to this mitzvah after we look at the total theme of this parsha.

Parsha of Transition
Chukas is a parsha of transition. We are transitioning from the phase of wandering in the desert to a new stage. This ends the forty years of travel and begins the coming into Israel. The people who came out of Egypt have, for the most part, died. The Children of Israel, those born to the former slaves, will go into Israel.

In this parsha Miriam dies, Aaron dies and Moses is told by Hashem that he will die in the midbar, the desert. Moses will not go into Israel. This ends the forty-year period of wandering.

Forty
Forty is a significant number and appears many times in the Torah text. Forty days of rain. Forty years of traveling. Moses was forty days on Mount Sinai. The spies went for forty days to check out the new land. The number forty represents transition or change; the concept of renewal; a new beginning.

Interpretation of Mitzvahs
Let's look at the mitzvah of the red cow and try to consider an interpretation for "pure becoming impure" and "impure becoming pure." We know that sometimes the good is not so good, and the bad is not so bad. Things have a relative meaning based upon what else is going on. Water is good. Too much water and the ground can become eroded, the rivers can overflow. This sounds practical and reasonable. But be cautious. Too much reasoning can be dangerous, especially if the questioning is subtly derisive, as we saw in the Korach rebellion.

The chukim exist so that we accept each mitzvah as it is presented. This is written in Torah and Torah is written by God. If I thought that a man, maybe an ancient version of Shakespeare, wrote the Torah, would I adhere to his commandment not to mix milk and meat? Why? Not unless the author could prove to me it was good for my health.
Rabbi Samson Raphael Hirsch interprets that the laws of purity and impurity are designed to sensitize man to his moral freedom whenever he is challenged by physical limitations. The red cow is structured to help man regain his equilibrium after a close encounter with death. When Jewish people go to a cemetery, upon leaving we wash our hands, to get the "death" off us. And so these rules are to rid us of the death that surrounds us.

Speak to the Rock
Miriam dies in this parsha. The well of Miriam brought water to the people. With her death there is no water. God said to Moses, "Take the staff...and speak to the rock." Moses took the staff and instead of speaking to the rock, he hit the rock. Moses lost his temper.

Anger
The worst trait is the trait of anger. When we are angry, we lose our mind. When we act in anger, we are not acting with reason. Maimonides said that with most middos (behavior traits), one finds the middle of the road. Take patience: we could have lots of patience and nothing happens, or too little patience and we are always pushing. A midpoint gives us balance, enough patience to give others time to act and give us time to think things through.

Anger has no midpoint. When we get angry, we are not ourselves anymore. A little bit of anger seems to accumulate into much anger. One can start with a difference of opinion, then lose himself and build into an angry exchange with the other person. Let it continue and it can blow into very aggressive and unbecoming behavior and reason is gone.

When Moses hit the rock, he functioned from anger. This behavior distances us from God. Knowledge leaves. Very angry people have a low level of functioning. We don't want to be with them. We can feel dirt coming from a person who is wild with anger. Intelligence is not ruling and the person is acting like an impulsive beast. Anger and ego are the two worst middos.

Was Moses Angry with the Rock?
Think about how many times the people came to Moses asking for something. Here they were, coming again. They had been through forty years of Hashem providing for them. Why would the people think that because Miriam was dead, there would be no water and they would all die of thirst?

Moses was just as illogical because he lost reason. Moses had everything provided for him for the forty years just as the people had. Perhaps the proper response could have been to remind the people that Hashem has provided for us all these years, he will provide water for us now. We had water before and we will have water now.

Yoga—Transition

The generation of the spies, the generation of Korach, and the generation of slavery: they all died off. The children of that generation, along with a new leader, Joshua, transitioned to the going into Israel.

Our yoga pose is a pose of transition.
Transition from being seated cross-legged to forming a tabletop with our bodies.
Sit on mat, cross-legged.
Rock forward to knees which are still crossed.
Hands on ground in front of you.
Uncross legs to create a tabletop.

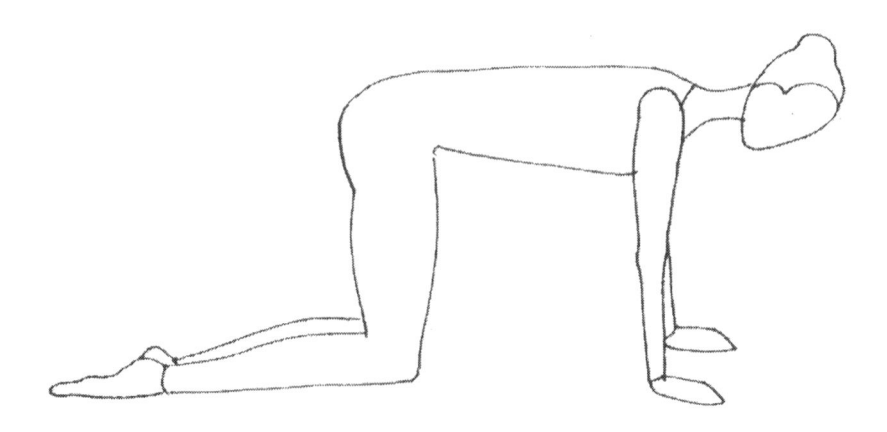

Balak (The Destroyer)

Parsha Insight — Man on a mission

Balak the Instigator
This is story of Bilam, but the parsha is called Balak. Balak is the king of Moab and the one who persuaded Bilam to curse the Jews. Balak is the instigator who set the action of this parsha into motion.

The discussions between Balak and Bilam happen without any Jews present. If it wasn't in Torah, we would not have known it occurred. Balak was afraid that the Jews were very powerful and concerned that if the Jews warred with his nation, the Jews would win. Balak wanted a sorcerer to curse the Jews.

A Happening
Balak asked Bilam to curse the Jews so that they would no longer be strong. Bilam has prophecy and he gets messages from God. Wait a minute! I thought Moses was an exception. He is. Moses talked to God face-to-face. Bilam talks to God at night, in the dark, as if it is a dream. God called Moses, God speaks to Moses. With Bilam, God happened upon Bilam. It was as though they sort of ran into each other. God did not go out of His way, it just happened.

Bilam, with his prophecy and his sorcerer's skills, thought he could find a wedge in God's ways to curse the Jews. He let God know that this was what he was going to do. God told Bilam, "You shall not go with them." Bilam then told Balak's people that he could not go with them because "Hashem refused to give me permission to go with you."

Balak sent another envoy out to Bilam and Bilam asked God again if he could go with them. God told him that if you really want to go, go, but the only thing that will come out of your mouth is what I let come out of your mouth. Bilam went on his mission to curse the Jews.

Man on a Mission

Bilam was so intent on cursing the Jews that he saddled up his own donkey. This is like the president of the United States checking the oil in the presidential limo. It was very unusual for Bilam to attend to the saddling of his donkey, but he was so possessed that he attended to all the details for his mission.

Bilam and the donkey are traveling when the donkey veers off the path after seeing an angel sent by God. Bilam, all wrapped up in his mission of hate, had tunnel vision and could not see the angel.

Bilam hits the donkey. The donkey presses into a wall and injures Bilam's leg. Bilam hits the donkey again and yet again. The donkey turns to Bilam and says, "What have I done to you that you struck me these three times?" Bilam gets into a conversation with the donkey. Bilam is so caught up in the mission and his anger that he loses all reason. When one is angry, judgment is lost. He is talking to the donkey and doesn't even notice how strange this is.

Consider us driving up Preston Road with all the construction at LBJ Expressway in Dallas. Nothing is moving and our car says, "You should have gone up Hillcrest" and we say, "Yeah, I know. Remind me next time" (told by a rabbi in Dallas, TX). You have to have lost your mind if you are talking to donkeys or cars.

Mission Impossible

Finally Bilam gets to where he is going. Bilam opens his mouth to curse the Jews and out comes a blessing. His mouth is doing what God wants, not what Bilam wants. God had warned Bilam that he would only be able to speak what God let him speak. Bilam has no control over his mouth. Just like his mind left him when he spoke to the donkey, now his mouth leaves him. Bilam's mission was becoming an impossible mission. Bilam was not stepping back, he was not asking, "Why am I being thwarted?"

Let us now look at how this parsha relates to our lives. Did you ever have a mission, something you felt you had to do, and whichever way you turned, it went wrong? You are blocked. You are desirous to make this happen—insistent that it should happen; and yet obstacles keep coming at you in all different directions. At that point you have a choice. You can say "When the going gets tough, the tough get going," and keep pushing ahead. Or, you could stop and ask, "How come it is so hard for me to do this? Maybe I need to step back and evaluate if this is where I should be."

On a bad project, someplace we should not be, hindrances come at us constantly. This is a signal that the project needs rethinking or that energies should be diverted to a more productive avenue. This does not mean that we should not work hard for something, it just means that we should be sure that our efforts are not misdirected.

When there is something we are supposed to do, when it is the right thing for us, things fall into place. If the activity will promote the kind of experience and event that we need, it happens. It goes well. We are comfortable. We may have some obstacles, but they are not insurmountable.

Nothing Happened
At the end of the parsha, Bilam and Balak meet up. It is as if they say "How do you do?" and they each go their separate ways.

So what happened? Nothing! All that conniving and planning and devious thoughts and actions, came to nothing. Bilam may have had prophecy, he may have been a sorcerer, but without God's allowing something to happen, nothing happens.

Lead-In to Next Parsha

People do not have downfalls because someone cursed them. Most downfalls occur because of the person's own actions. If we look at the things where we were not successful, it wasn't because someone cursed us, it was because we inadvertently made it happen. We made the wrong choices. We decided incorrectly. We interpreted wrongly. We had make-believe plans that we never firmed up. We are all guilty of this.

At the very end of this parsha, the Jewish men engaged in immoral behavior with the Midianite and Moabite women. They did not honor their vows to modesty or morality. They prayed to idols. One of the men took one of the Midianite women and, in front of Moses' tent, had sexual relations.

Pinchas saw this and was horrified. He took a spear and pierced the two of them. The zealous action of Pinchas stopped a plague that had already killed 24,000 Jews. Bilam's desire to curse the Jews came to naught. The Jews had brought a plague on themselves with their own actions. Without God's allowing something to happen, nothing happens.

Midrashim are analogies to enhance the story. There is a midrash that Bilam cursed the Jews and that created the immorality. Parsha Balak tells us that we are responsible for our own actions and that the outcome rests on our own shoulders. We have free choice and there is accountability for what subsequently happens. We cannot put the blame on someone else; the charge rests on ourselves.

Yoga—Donkey

Start in tabletop pose.
Go to downward dog.
Bend your knees and arms a bit.
Bring your right leg into your chest, breathe in.
Kick out and back with right leg, breathe out.
Change so that your left leg does the kicking.

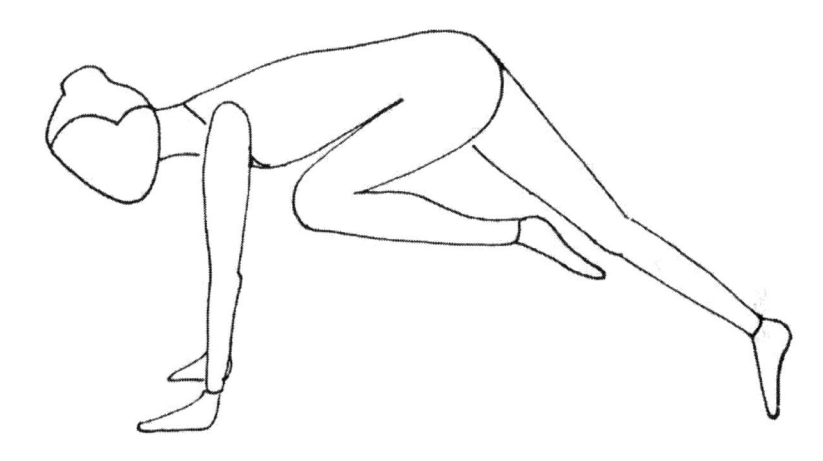

Pinchas (dark-skinned)

Parsha Insight — Zealous

A Kohen Forever
Last week's parsha ended with Pinchas, a spear, and a man and a woman shish-kabobed. Pinchas' actions were due to his zealousness. He was dedicated to punishing immoral behavior so defiantly sinful that it was right in front of Moses' tent. A Midianite woman and a Prince of the Jews committing an immoral act in public. This outward display of sinful immorality and people worshiping idols brought on a plague. Pinchas stopped the plague — but not before twenty-four thousand people had died.

God rewarded Pinchas for his zealousness because the act was done to avenge God. Pinchas became a Kohen, a priest in the Temple. He did not only become a Kohen, he became a Kohen Gadol, which is the high priest. The hereditary Kohen status passed down not just from Pinchas to his male children but to all of his future generations. This is a wonderful reward that God gave Pinchas.

The parsha tells us that Pinchas is the son of Elazar, who is the son of Aaron. We know that the sons of Aaron are Kohanim. Doesn't that mean that Pinchas was already a Kohen? When Aaron and his sons became Kohanim, Hashem said that all subsequently born males from the line of Aaron would be Kohanim. At that time Pinchas had already been born, so he was not included in the "subsequently born" category. Also, he was a grandson of Aaron, not a son. So Pinchas missed out on being a Kohen but he was a Levi. He was left out when Aaron, his sons, and those subsequently born to those sons were declared Kohanim. Hashem righted this when Pinchas showed his zealousness and his willingness to avenge God's honor.

No Permission to Be a Zealot

One thing we have to be very careful about. The parsha goes into this, but not completely. It skirts around the issue and says, if in the heat of the moment you get carried away and the purpose is not for your gain and only to avenge God, then zealousness is okay. But if you have to stop and ask someone, shall I avenge God by killing these people, then the answer is no. Nobody is going to tell you to go ahead and do it.

Much in Torah has to do with law. Lawyers, even non-Jewish lawyers, love to read Torah. So many of our laws come from Torah. Torah does not want to say, go ahead and be zealous and become a vigilante and take on the judgment and the execution by yourself.

The Daughters Get the Property

Another interesting part in this parsha has to do with the five daughters of Zelophehad. He died with no sons. At that time, the father's property was passed on to sons and not to daughters. The five women went to Moses and said that their father died without sons. If his inheritance did not come to the five of them, then it wouldn't be in the family anymore. It would go to distant relatives. They asked that the inheritance stay in the family. The lineage of their father went all the way back to Yaakov, so it was very important to the daughters that the property stay with the family.

Imagine in current times. My father died with two daughters, no sons. It would have been an injustice if my sister and I would not inherit. Moses took this to Hashem and Hashem said that the daughters were right. They should inherit their father's estate.

Leadership Training

Moses has already found out that he will not be allowed to go into Israel. He will die before the Jews enter Israel. He needs a successor. Torah is very descriptive of Moses' leadership role and how to appoint and train a successor. It is brilliant in understanding people and leadership.

Appoint your successor before you die (retire or take another job).
Have a plan of succession.
Train your successor in all the things for which he is responsible.
Train him not just in Torah and laws (rules and regulations). Train him in demeanor and the way to deal with people.
Make sure that the people know that he is the chosen successor so that they willingly accept him.

We saw that Joshua has spirit. In the story of the spies, Moses prayed for Joshua because Joshua had an impetuous nature. He might get angry at people before he thought it all out. Joshua did not have the patience of Caleb (the other positive-speaking spy) and he might have pressed his point too much. Now Moses has to train Joshua how to hold back a little bit, to be quiet, to get the whole story, and to speak when the timing is right.

It is very obvious that Joshua will not be Moses' equal. Moses had a glow on his face like the sun, and Joshua was like the moon, a reflection of Moses. This means that Joshua stood in front of Moses and learned from him.

Yom Tovim (holidays) and Shabbos
The Yom Tovim of Rosh Chodesh, the three festivals of Pesach, Shavuos, and Succos, Shemini Atzeres which comes immediately after Succos, Rosh Hashanah, and Yom Kippur are mentioned along with Shabbos. These holidays were all introduced earlier in the Torah. Why are they repeated now? We are passing on leadership, passing on Shabbos and holidays to a new administration. The importance must be seen and understood. Shabbos is mentioned along with the holidays, even though it occurs every week. This is because Shabbos is so crucial to Jews that it deserves to be part of the Yom Tovim.

Yoga—Camel

We have been schlepping around the desert for forty years and haven't seen a camel.
I feel bad that we have not yet done the camel pose.

Starts on your knees, hip width apart.
Your hands are on your back hips, fingers pointing downward.
Your palms are over your kidneys.
Lean back as far as you can.
If you can hold your heels, go ahead.
Practice along the edge of the bed or a sofa for security.

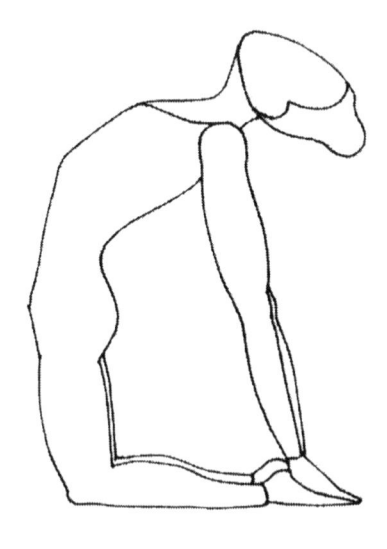

Mattos (tribes)
Masei (journeys of)

Parsha Insight — Fear of the unknown

The Three Weeks
Mattos-Masei is always read between the 17th of Tamuz and the 9th of Av. These are "the three weeks," and historically bad things happened during these three weeks. During the Roman war against the Jews, the 17th of Tamuz was when the walls of Jerusalem were broken and the 9th of Av is when the Temple was destroyed. The 9th of Av is especially ominous.

The ten spies came back with a bad report on the 9th of Av.
The first Temple was destroyed on the 9th of Av.
The second Temple was destroyed on the 9th of Av.
The final massacre of the bar Kochba rebellion against Rome was on the 9th of Av.
The last day Jews were permitted in Spain during the Spanish Inquisition was in 1492 on the 9th of Av.
World War I started on the 9th of Av.
Hitler's proclamation to kill the Jews was on the 9th of Av.
(History from Chabad.org)

Vows
This is a period of mourning and, spiritually, we are uncomfortable. The notes from Chabad.org show the many terrible occurrences on the 9th of Av. Can it get any worse than what we have already experienced?

The parsha's opening sentences are about vows. Vows are things you say, such as "I'll never drink again" or "I'll never smoke again." During these three weeks a lot of people feel that if they make a vow, that they will be able to prevent a bad event. If it were only so simple. Wouldn't it be nice if the power was in my hands and if I did this, then God will or will not let something else happen?

If you were the type of person to make a vow, this would be the time that you would be most susceptible. There is a category of people who make vows, called nazir. Making vows is not encouraged. Most vows are made in the moment, and perhaps one is not thinking clearly of all its implications.

The three weeks are a period of sadness and fear. A person gets caught up in this and wants to do something to control the situation so that nothing bad happens. So he takes a vow.

Vows of Married Women and Young Girls
Once you take a vow, to annul it you have to go before a beit din, a Jewish rabbinic court. A young girl and a married woman can have their vows voided by their father or husband. The wife cannot annul her husband's vow. The husband can annul his wife's vow only if it affects the marriage. The father can annul his young daughter's vow, because she was too young to be aware of the implications of the vow. The annulment must be upon hearing of it. If the father or husband hears about the vow and does nothing, it stands.

Segula
A segula is a procedure that is not based on any logic yet is believed to be effective in changing a situation or protecting a person from harm. For example, if I light a candle and say a prayer for forty days, then my house will sell or I will make a good shiddoch (a marriage arrangement).

I have to admit that several years ago, another woman and I made a segula by lighting a candle and praying for each other for forty days. We each had a house to sell and needed to effect the sale because it was causing a great financial strain. After the forty days, within two weeks, we each had viable contracts on our houses. Don't ask me to explain it. Praying works and praying for someone else works better.

War against the Midianites
Hashem spoke to Moses saying, "Take vengeance for the Children of Israel against the Midianites." This is a call to go to war against the Midianites. Hashem told Moses to take vengeance for the benefit of Moses and the people. After the war, Moses should prepare for his death. If Moses told the people he would die after the war, they would not fight. So Moses told the people to go against the Midianites to inflict "Hashem's vengeance." Moses changed the wording from his taking revenge to Hashem's taking revenge, reasoning that the people would fight for Hashem's vengeance even if that meant that Moses' life would end after the war.

War with Armies and War with Yetzer Hora
The reason for the Midianite war and the vengeance was because of the immoral and enticing Midianite women. The Israelites killed all the adult male Midianites, but the soldiers did not kill the women and children. Moses got very angry and said that the women were the ones who started this whole trouble. All the adult women needed to die. The officers got very upset and said, "Not a man of us is missing." This means that not only had no man died, but no man was induced to leave his army and go with the Midianite women.

There were two wars being fought. The outside war of armies (determined by Hashem) and the internal war decided by each man dealing with his yetzer hora, his evil inclination. Man was fighting his evil inclination and deciding what was right and what was wrong.

We Will Stay in Jordan
In Chapter 32 Gad and Reuben request to stay on this side of Jordan River and not go into Israel. They said, "We have a lot of cattle and this is good land. We could raise our cattle over here." When Moses heard this he repeated, "You are not going into Israel, you are not going to help us gain the land, you are going to stay back." They replied, "Yes, we will go into Israel and fight and then we will come back across the Jordan to our land." Moses said, "Where are your priorities? First you will take care of your animals and then your children and women." They then said, "We will take care of our children first, then our wives, and then our animals. We will go and fight with you and then we will come back to our land." Here we see the art of negotiation, with lots of give and take.

But what are they doing? They are on the edge of the Jordan River. They have been wandering for forty years. Across the river is Israel and yet they decide, before even going into Israel, "Let's stay here." They knew that the land of Israel was for them, that it was good land. Why were they so impatient? Why make a premature decision without even seeing if the land of Israel could accommodate their cattle? After all these years of going towards settling in Israel, it seems preposterous that they are right in front of the goal, and they back off.

Fear of the Unknown
Do we do this? Fear of change. Fear of the unknown is paralyzing and sometimes the unknown is success. You see this in business: a company struggles for years to be successful, they are just on the edge of making it big, and they do the stupidest thing—buy the worst inventory, make a dumb investment, change a policy, and avoid success. Self-sabotage. Stopping ourselves before the success. Imagine forty years of working towards something, you and your children and your parents before you. You get to the edge of making it, and stop.

Naming the Places

In the parsha Massei, Moses summarizes the forty-year journey by naming all the places the Jewish Nation camped. Since these places were not existing towns, the names that Moses gave described the incidents that occurred at the locations.

Yoga–Walk

Last week's camel is loaded and there is no room for us to ride. We have to walk beside it.

Like walking the dog in downward dog, only we are upright.
Lift heel and keep toes on ground;
First right heel, then left.
Walking in place.
Breathe, long inhales and long exhales.
Loosens the knees and hips.

Book V

Devarim/Deuteronomy

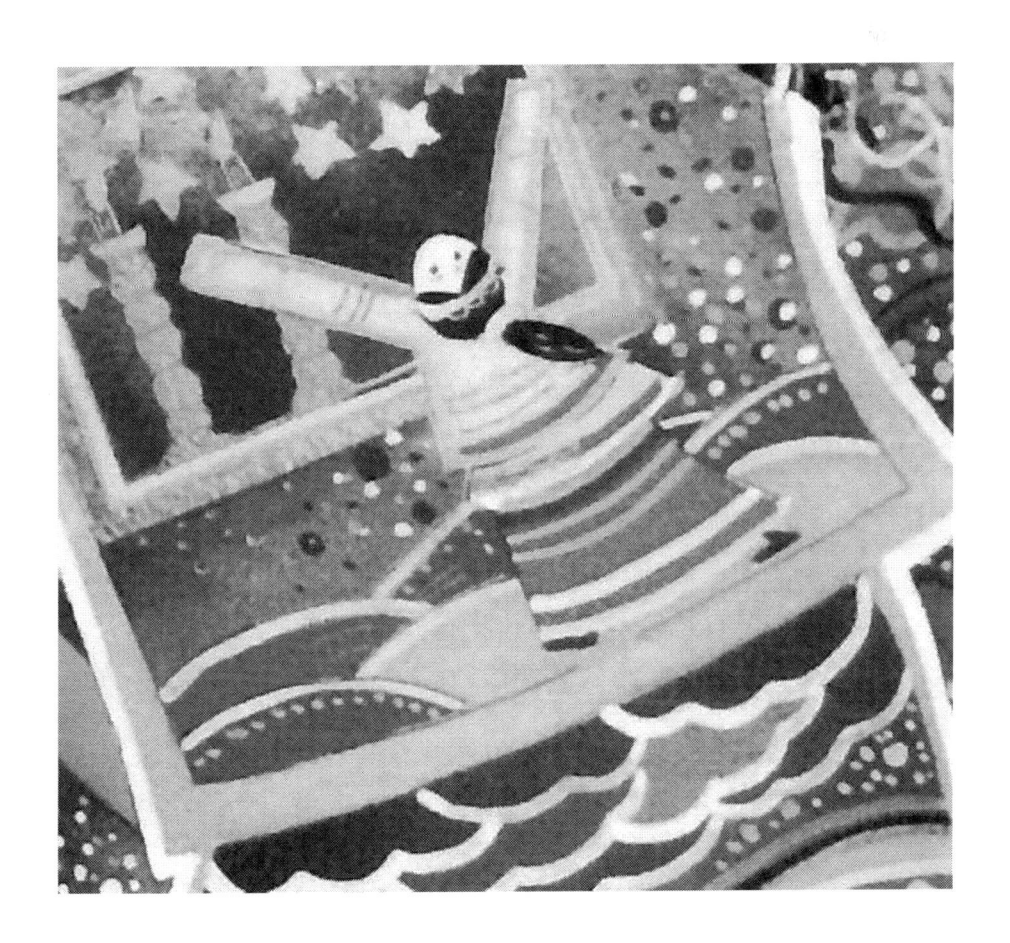

Devarim (words)

Parsha Insight — Loving rebuke

A Book of Loving Rebuke
The book of Devarim represents the last five weeks of Moses' life. The Jewish people have not entered Israel and are at the banks of the Jordan River. Moses is giving the people guidance, discipline, and constructive criticism.

Moses Is Speaking
Moses begins, "These are the words that Moses spoke to all Israel." At this point, Moses is speaking. God had spoken to him but these are Moses' words. In prior parshas the words were Hashem's and we are told "Hashem spoke to Moses." In Devarim, Moses says, "Hashem spoke to me." The book, Devarim, is from the mouth of Moses. Moses spoke to everybody. He did not just call the leaders, he spoke to everyone at the same time because he wanted to make sure that everyone heard all he had to say.

The message that Moses expressed was that for forty years Hashem took care of you and you lacked nothing. Be happy with your lot. Trust in Hashem. Have no jealousies. Have peace of mind. Moses said this so that the people would look back over forty years and realize that they were well taken care of. Yes, they were coming to something new; but they had been taken care of in the past and they would be taken care of in the future.

These are the words that Moses spoke to all of Israel. The events occurring at the sites where they camped are only implied. The mention of the places invoked the memories of the people. This is a gentle rebuke for their past sins and discord.

"On the other side of Jordan concerning the wilderness." The wilderness is the desert and they did not starve in the desert although there had been complaints that they would starve in the desert.

"Concerning the Araba" — the Midonites — "and opposite the Sea of Reeds," which was where they complained that Moses brought them out of Egypt to the Sea to be drowned. The Egyptians were bearing down behind them and the Sea was in front of them. The people cried that Moses brought them here to die.

"Between Paran" — the sins of the spies — and "Tophel and Lavan" — where is the meat? They wanted meat and were not satisfied with the manna. "and Hazaroth" — the rebellion of Korach. All these places were given names in the prior parsha but now they are referred to as a reminder of how the people acted.

"and DiZahab" is where the sin of the Golden Calf occurred.

This is a subtle rebuke; instead of harshly detailing the event and the negative behavior of the people, the places are just named. Most people, when subtly told about the inappropriate things they did, can appreciate the lesson. Honorable people are aware of their actions. They just need a gentle and loving admonition to see their errors and learn from them.

Moses is teaching as a tender and devoted father. We are on the other side of the Jordan and coming to Israel. Look back and see that God took care of you before and will take care of you again.

This is good advice for each of us. Look at where we are today. We have lived through difficulties and learned from our experiences. We have traveled the road of the past till now. We came to this point and we will go forward with the confidence that we will be able to handle the future.

Yoga—Sore feet

After all that walking, and now standing on the other side of Jordan, let's give our feet a treat.

Take a tennis ball and roll it back and forth on bare feet.
Roll side to side.
Roll up and down.
Press down on heel and press down on ball of feet.
Ahh!

This is a great foot massage.

Va'eschanan (And I besought)

Parsha Insight — Remember and safeguard

Moses Implored Hashem
Moses spoke to all the people: leaders, men, women, and children gathered together. Moses is transferring leadership of the nation to Joshua, and he wants to make sure that the people know what is expected of them. The Torah's meanings and the people's understandings were crucial. Moses knew he was not going to go into Israel, and the parsha opens with "I implored Hashem." Moses was saying, to paraphrase, "My Lord, please let me go into Israel."

Midrash
There is a midrash (a parallel or a story) that says that Moses prayed five hundred and fifteen times to Hashem. Imploring — which implies that I know that maybe I don't deserve it but, please — begging Hashem to allow him to enter Israel. Hashem then told Moses, "Don't ask me anymore because if you ask me one more time, I might have to let you go." Wait a minute! That sounds like a good thing: let me ask one more time and I'll get what I want. But sometimes there are things we should not do, places we don't need to be. We might be begging, pleading, praying, hoping it comes to pass, but Hashem does not give it to us. Hashem knows better than we do.

Ask one more time and Hashem says, "Okay, you think you know better — go ahead — do"; even though it may not be best. You want it enough? Okay. Free choice. According to midrash, Moses did not ask again.

Why Could Moses Not Go Into Israel?

Some say Moses was prohibited from entering Israel because he hit the rock. Why did he hit the rock? He did so because he was very angry with the Jewish people. They made him angry with their continuous requests, especially since they were requests that showed a lack of faith in God. Now it's the water, before it was the meat; before that they thought they would die in the desert and before that they thought they would drown. It was always something else. Moses got so angry.

When we get angry, we lose our mind and act in negative ways. Moses hit the rock out of anger and frustration. Moses allowed his anger to overcome him; and that is why Hashem did not let him go into Israel. It was not because he hit the rock but the reason why he hit the rock.

When people get angry, they lose their head and do things that are not in their best interest. This is a lesson to the people about what happens when you let your temper control you. We are responsible for the consequences of our actions.

Do Not Add or Subtract from Torah

Moses tells the people that we do not change anything in Torah. We don't add to Torah and we certainly don't subtract to make it more comfortable and to our liking. Even if we don't follow Torah 100%, we are not saying that Torah is to be changed. We know what we are doing and we acknowledge that we are doing things as we wish and not as Hashem wishes.

Remember and Safeguard

The Ten Commandments are now repeated with lessons of how to follow them. In Exodus it says remember the Sabbath. To remember the Sabbath is to sanctify it, to make it holy, to separate the Sabbath from the rest of the week.

In this parsha, it says "Safeguard the Sabbath day." Safeguarding is different from remembering. To safeguard is to protect. Protect by not doing certain things. You refrain from work, you refrain from driving, you safeguard to protect and make holy.

"You shall remember the Sabbath": these are the positive things to do, the active things to do to make the Sabbath holy. "Make Shabbos": these are the things you will do to sanctify Shabbos. The time you light the Shabbos candles is the time that you make the Shabbos. We buy special foods for Shabbos. It is always fun to have a special treat of foods that we usually do not have during the week. I'm partial to dessert and I look for a nice parve (not meat and not dairy) cake or cookies for Shabbos. This separates the Shabbos from the rest of the week. We set the table a little fancier for Shabbos. I like eating in the dining room rather than the kitchen on Shabbos.

Yoga—Protect and enhance

We safeguard
We protect ourselves.
Precautionary measures to take in yoga.
Do only the positions that you are comfortable doing; stretch your practice but don't do anything outside your comfort zone. I can't stand on my head and I don't even try it.
Don't go as far if it hurts.
Watch your body.
Yoga is not a competitive sport.
Do not race through yoga practice.

We remember
We enhance
Listen to yoga audio and actively try to improve your posture.
Hold a position a little longer.
Breathe more fully and hold a bit at the top and the bottom of your inhales and exhales.

Eikev (this word means because and also means heel)

Parsha Insight — Fear

"The entire commandment that I command you today you shall observe..." Hashem wants us to know that we are to follow all of the mitzvahs and not just some of them. This parsha is about our actions and the consequences. Heel means to follow. Mind me. Observe and follow my ways. Stay close by me. "Because" if you do this, then this will follow.

Fear Him
Chapter 8:6 of this parsha is difficult to understand. "You shall observe the commandments of Hashem, your God, to go in His ways and to fear Him." I always get distraught about fearing God. And so many other women have said the same thing to me. I understand love and awe. But fear; fear terrifies me.

I didn't really understand what fearing God meant until I came across this explanation in the book *Living Each Week* by Rabbi Abraham J. Twerski M.D.

A loving father tells a child, "Don't go out in the road, you will get hurt. If I see you stepping off the curb to go out in the road, I am going to punish you. I will take away your privileges. I will take away your treats." The kid then is afraid of the father. Years go by and the now adult child comes to the understanding that the father was afraid that his child would get hurt by a car and so he made threats to get his child's attention. The father wanted to make sure that his child obeyed. Dad wanted to be sure to implant danger in his child's mind. The child thinks the fear is of the father because he will bring the punishment. As the child matures, he knows that it is the cars and trucks that create the hazardous event. The father is only trying to protect his child.

Every one of the mitzvahs is for our own good. We are told the laws of kosher and the laws of purity. We are to follow these laws for our good. If there is punishment, it is because of the inherent element or the underlying purpose in the mitzvah. That is what brings the punishment, and that is the fearful thing. It is the commandment that I have not followed that is going to hurt me. Inherent in eating non-kosher food is the attachment to non-Jewish ways, which leads one away from a Torah life.

Hashem gives us everything. The parsha recaps. Chapter 10:12 again says, "O Israel, what does Hashem, your God, ask of you? Only to fear Hashem, your God, to go in His ways and to love Him. ..."

Rashi says that this is where we exercise our free choice. We can go in His ways and love Him and only have to fear Hashem. We won't have to fear life. What is God asking of us? We are only asked to fear Hashem. This is the one thing that God does not control. We have the free choice to fear or not to fear God. To love or not to love God. To have awe and respect for Hashem or not. Rashi sees everything else in Hashem's hands. Once we stop paying attention to what Hashem says, whether we call that attention fear, awe, or love; at that point, we suffer the consequences. We each have to look at our actions, consider the consequences and make a decision.

This is from the Lubavitcher Rebbe of Chabad: "Within every love, there is fear: The fear of separation from that which you love." What do you fear? If you fear not having enough money, then you love the material world. If you fear what she said and how she looked at you, then you love the social world. If you love Hashem, then there is no room for fear in this world.

This is from Rabbi Jeffrey Wolfson Goldwasser from Judaism.about.com: "Fear of God can't mean to be incapacitated or run screaming because that would take or keep you away from God." We translate "yirah" into "awe" of God so that we do not have the anxious fears that contribute to dread or loathing. We know the divine presence is with us at all times.

We come to an understanding that life has meaning. We have startling awareness that the choices we make have consequences. A Jew fears God by accepting God's divine presence around us all the time. If we fear God this way, we can never say, "It does not matter how I behave in this circumstance because no one will ever know."

This is what Moses was teaching the Children of Israel. Fear of God is one of the six hundred and thirteen mitzvahs. All the other mitzvahs are included in Fear of God because it makes all of them meaningful. Moses is saying that without fear of God, the mitzvahs are a burden instead of an act of love and a way to get closer to God.

The Shema
The Shema is a prayer that tells us that our acts will bring about certain consequences. When we look at the Shema, we see that the first part is singular and the second part is plural.
Rashi says that this is about miracles. Miraculous miracles, positive or negative, do not happen to an individual. They happen to the general population. If God is going to make a flood, he does not do a flood for only one person with everybody else dry. The Red Sea did not part for one, all the waters parted. A miraculous act—not within the realms of everyday—is not for one, it is for all. We all saw it. Everyone was involved. Someone did not get the idea in the middle of the night. Everyone saw the Red Sea split. Everyone got Hashem's words at Mount Sinai.

The first part of the Shema is about us as an individual. The second part of the Shema is about us as a community.

Yoga—Chair pose

Just like in life, in yoga we have to work through fear. We fear that our body might not do what we want it to do. We need to see our strengths. Let's do the chair pose and get past the fear of falling.

Chair pose
Hold your arms straight out.
Feet hip width apart.
Raise arms and bend down and back as if sitting in a chair.
Hold. You won't fall.
Back does arch.
Balance keeps you in place.

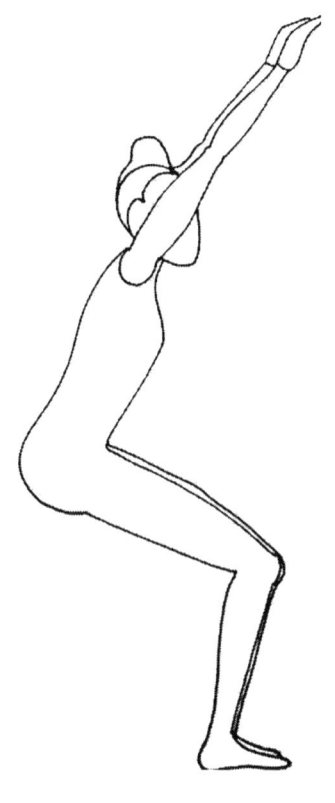

Re'eh (see; before you)

Parsha Insight – Responsibility

In the Hebrew, "see" (re'eh) is singular, while "before you" (lifneichem) is plural

"See, I present before you today, a blessing and a curse." Moses is saying this to each of the people as individuals, "See," the individual you. Each and every separate person. Then, "I present before you today," plural. I'm speaking to all of you; the people of Israel. Follow the mitzvahs and there will be blessings. Stray and follow the gods of others and there will be curses.

"See," singular you, the individual, make the choice. This is your free choice. Last week we said that you have the free choice to fear Hashem. You decide to do the mitzvahs because you fear God, or you are in awe of God. You choose to do the mitzvahs because you know that it is the proper thing to do.

As a group of people, "I present before you," everybody, y'all (in Texas). You as an individual count for yourself and also as a representative of the Jews. You are a component of the Jewish people. A convert has to be willing to be part of all the Jews and to accept all the things that being Jewish means. At the base of Mount Sinai, at the time of the revelation, all the people said, "We are here." They accepted being part of the nation of Jews and accepted the Torah.

When we are part of a group, we have a responsibility to the group. The perspective of the group influences the individual and the behavior of the group influences us. Think about the people who are closest to us, those we spend the most time with. We are the average of the people with whom we surround ourselves. If we choose to be in a close religious group, study together, have Shabbos dinners with each other, send our children to the same schools, we behave as they do. The norm for the group is established and we are in the group because we are comfortable in their presence. Their morals match ours. We realize that if we did anything really awful, the group would be embarrassed by our actions. Our behavior would reflect upon the group. We are a representative of the groups with whom we identify.

Not only are we considerate of our actions and their impact on the group, we are concerned about the group's standing in the larger community. If the group is seen as highly respected and as movers and shakers of the city, for example, we are proud to be part of this group. If the group takes an unpopular and detrimental position on a topic or situation, we have a responsibility to voice our opinion and try to lead the group in a more positive direction. We are committed to use our influence for the common good. Rabbi Shlomo Luntschitz (1550-1619; in his Torah commentary "Kli Yakar") says each individual should feel an obligation to the group.

Meat
Before this parsha, meat was only eaten when it was sacrificed. Since the people were in the midbar (desert) and they had the mishkan (tabernacle) with them, sacrificial offerings were able to be made in the sanctuary. You shared the food with your family and friends. You shared your thankfulness.

When the people would settle in Israel, they would be living far away from the Temple and so they were given permission to schecht meat (ritually slaughter) at locations away from the Temple. The people had a hunger for meat and in this parsha, they were given permission to eat meat even when not for sacrificial purposes when in Israel and when dispersed over great distances.

...Shall Not Eat the Blood
There was a warning that went with this permission to eat meat: do not violate the prohibition of blood. What does this mean? We were already told not to eat blood. What is the purpose of saying it again now? Just because we have permission to eat meat, we cannot eat without restraints. Someone eating meat with blood dripping conjures up pictures of gluttony. Remember the movie "Tom Jones" and the character was eating with both hands, with food stuff dripping from his mouth? Nice! We think of overindulgence with food as greed: no restraints on physical desires.

Gluttony leads to sin. The "Sefer HaChinuch," published anonymously in 13th century Spain, tells us that Israel "grew fat and rebelled." This is saying that when a person is overstuffed and complacent, he's more inclined to turn his back on God. The 13th century author is saying that as time went on, Israel (the Jews) got so comfortable and so interested in satisfying physical desires that they left no room for God.

The Rambam wrote that gluttony is bad for one's health, and that which is physically harmful is spiritually destructive as well. So, even though something is permitted and we are encouraged to enjoy and be happy, we must control ourselves and put restraints on our passions. This warning about not violating the prohibition of blood is a warning about eating without restraint. Do not overindulge. It is also a caution about any behavior without restraint and the importance of being in control of ourselves.

Out-of-Control Behavior

We see children with out-of-control behavior. They have a temper tantrum, falling down on the ground, kicking and screaming. They want something and have learned negative ways to attract adult attention to get what they want. They need boundaries and it is the responsibility of the adults around the child to provide them.

Adults with out-of-control behavior and mental problems scream and cry and hit and throw things. Not very different from the little child. They name-call and blame others. They intimidate and are cruel. They insist that their viewpoint is the only one that matters. Mature individuals learn self-control and restraint. We censor ourselves and do not hurt others. We postpone gratification and think about the other person.

We need to be in control of our behavior and watch what we are doing. Out-of-control behavior may be caused by too much stress. If we want something and we want it now and are not immediately satisfied, stress develops. We can feel so much pressure that we get nervous. We are not making good decisions. All the stress causes us to become egocentric. We concentrate so much on me, myself, and I that there is no room for anyone else. This kind of behavior promotes greed, anger and selfishness.

Yoga—Happy baby

Yoga can help you to be calm and to focus on one issue at a time. Too many of us are multitasking and putting too much pressure on ourselves. Concentrate and relax with your yoga practice.

Very important in yoga is proper breathing. Breathe slowly and fully, inhaling and exhaling through your nose. Pay attention to your body and visualize each part of you in the pose.

Our pose for this parsha is the happy baby. You smile just thinking about holding your legs up, your hands holding your ankles (or your feet), and rocking gently side to side. Everything is good. You have everything you need. Put a smile on your face. This is such a fun pose that you will reduce stress by having a good time.

Happy baby
Lie on your back on the floor with your legs up and knees wide.
Bend your knees and bring them towards the floor.
Flex your feet to ceiling and hold your feet at the instep.
Rock gently side to side, massaging your hips and back.

When you are finished, to get up from the ground, bring your knees to the right side.
Turn slowly to the right side.
Use both hands to push yourself up.
This is a good way to get out of bed.
You won't feel light-headed.

Shoftim (judges)

Parsha Insight — Wholeheartedness

Three Branches of Government
"Judges and officers shall you appoint for yourself in all your cities." The Jewish people, upon returning to Israel after the Exodus from Egypt, had the mitzvah of appointing judges, officers and a melech (a king) "whom Hashem, your God, shall choose."

The United States of America has three branches of government, as established in the Constitution written in 1776. Ancient Greece and Rome had separation of powers. Did they get the idea from Torah?

Appoint for Yourself
Appoint judges and officers to uphold the laws for your community. Your duty is to obey the laws of the government and also to adhere to your own rules of conduct. Appoint yourself as judge and officer over your own actions. Be the one to monitor your behavior, set your boundaries, judge yourself and be responsible for the consequences of your actions. Be strict with yourself and uphold the laws that you set for yourself. The laws we wish others to follow are laws that apply to us as well.

Last week we learned that we will be blessed if we follow Torah and cursed if we violate Torah. Torah now gives us a judicial and an enforcement system for each city. To live as an honorable person, one takes responsibility for his actions. Rambam said in the "Rules of Repentance" (Hilchot Teshuva), "a person's status as righteous or evil is not predetermined. A person is fully deserving or culpable because he has the ability to choose to do right or to continue to do evil."

Rabbi Chanina taught: "Pray for the welfare of the government, for without fear of governmental authorities people would swallow each other alive" (Pirkei Avos 3:2). Justice must be righteous and not perverted. Judges may not take bribes and must treat all persons equally and with respect.

Perfection of Items
In the time of the Temple sacrifices, only perfect items could be brought to Hashem. No blemished animals or produce could be taken into the Temple for sacrifice. This maintains the integrity of the Temple. It is not fitting to bring your old, sick animals as a sacrifice. What are you sacrificing? The poor thing is close to death already.
You cannot use stolen items as a sacrifice nor can stolen objects can be used for a mitzvah. If you stole candlesticks would they be appropriate to use to light Shabbos candles? It is a high level of chutzpah (nerve) to bentch licht (light and bless the candles) if they were stolen. It is a perversion of justice. Mitzvahs must be done with proper objects.

The Jewish King
The king was chosen from among his people, and if someone rebelled against him, the act was punished by death. The king had to have the Torah with him at all times so that he remembered his place in this world and did not let the power over the people and their adoration of him go to his head. The Torah, in his possession, protects him from the negative character trait of arrogance. He might be king on earth, but Hashem is the true Melech.

The king should not have too many horses, too many wives, or too much money. The king needs to be told not to have too much, because it will taint him. We can see how people who value their money, their houses, and their cars too much can be arrogant. Torah warns us against behaviors that lead to arrogance.

Arrogance-The Worst Trait
Rabbi Yisroel Salanter, a very important mussar leader (school of character trait development), says that arrogance is the worse trait. A person who is arrogant is so revolting that when Rabbi Salanter sees this arrogant person, it makes him want to vomit.

Just as anger makes one lose his mind and have bad traits, arrogance does the same. When we are arrogant we have too much ego, we do not have humility, we have a sense of entitlement, and we get angry very quickly if things aren't just the way we want them.

An arrogant person has to make himself appear better than anyone else. He will have all the good ideas and will never listen to others. His interest is only in promoting himself. An arrogant person is overbearing and coercive and very unpleasant to be with. When he has disregard for others, he is truly evil.

Wholehearted Trust
"You shall be wholehearted with Hashem" 18:13. Wholeheartedness means that you have emuna (know that there is God) and bitochan (trust that all that occurs is because of God and for your ultimate good). You are consistent in your trust in God. At what point does your hishtadlus — your effort — come in to play?

We are talking about normal effort, not herculean acts. Here is an example: After class I will have dinner. I trust that there will be food for me to eat and that what I have to eat is for my good. I may not afford lamb chops, but I have fruit and vegetables and chopped meat in the refrigerator. Now my hishtadlus: Hashem has provided the ways and means for me to purchase these items. I had to work to earn money, I had to go to the grocery store to buy my food, and I have to cook it and serve it to me, so that I will have dinner. Normal effort. The food will not walk onto my plate (and if it does, I'm not going to eat it!).

We struggle with this daily. At what point do we trust in God and at what point does hishtadlus stop being "normal"? How much effort should we put into making something happen? At what point are we forcing the issue? When we force something, it is not really that good for us.

There was a point when we crossed over from normal to excessive. It is a fine line, but we probably recognized a change, a catch, a red flag that told us "pause." If it did not register, it was because we pushed it away. Learn to look for those signs and acknowledge them. They are coming to us for a reason. Perhaps it is instinct, or past knowledge, or Hashem telling us to stop, to know that if we are going past normal effort, and that maybe this is not for us.

Such a fine line. We want to use our potential, we want to be the best us we can be. Maybe the timing is not right. Maybe we need more information. Maybe we just need to pause and shore up our resources and try harder. This differs for each of us. Make for yourself a judge.

Yoga—Plank pose

The plank pose is a total body pose.
Being wholehearted is being totally involved.

Start position in tabletop pose.
On the ground, on your hands and knees.
Walk back till your legs are straight back.
Your arms are straight and your toes are on the ground.
This is the full plank on toes.
The half plank is when you are resting on your knees rather than your toes.
This pose will strengthen your muscles.

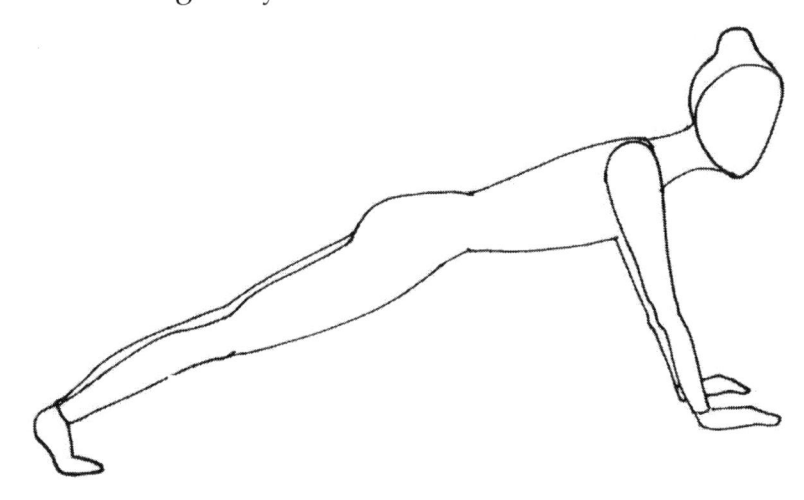

Ki Seitzei (when you go out)

Parsha Insight — Moral fiber

This parsha is a collection of mitzvahs, some given before and repeated here, and some new. These mitzvahs are value laws and not criminal laws. You would not go to jail for doing or not doing any of these laws. They are laws about one's moral fiber. Ignoring these laws means your core values are not up to par. They are ignored by people who live on the edge. These folks are not criminal but their behavior is not acceptable in society.

In wartime, soldiers' values are lax and they take advantage of women. This parsha tells the soldier to slow down his desires and not rush into anything.

If you have a firstborn son from your first wife, whom you divorced (Torah says you hated her), and then had a son from the favored wife, you do not dismiss your firstborn son. The firstborn, regardless of your care for your first wife, remains your firstborn son.

If we have a rebellious son, an incorrigible child, one whom we see having major behavior issues, the Torah says that he doesn't deserve to live. Subsequent writings have told us that it never came to pass that such a child was killed, but the law was there. Basically this is saying that parents must teach their children. When we see the first signs of erratic and damaging behavior, it is our job to train our child to improve and act differently. Don't say that he will grow out of it. Do something. Parents are afraid of their children. They want to be the child's friend. The child gets the wrong message. The child keeps upping the negative behavior looking for boundaries and the parents are not providing any. Let's face it, if destructive behavior by this child caused a terrible event on Tuesday, he wasn't so okay on Monday. It is the parent's obligation to stop the behavior as soon as they see it. The parents have to care for their children and teach them how to live in society.

Laws of divorce. It is better to divorce than to live in a house of hatefulness. Torah provides means for divorce. Hatefulness hurts the entire family: the husband and wife and the children.

A man should not wear women's clothing and a woman should not wear men's clothing.

You shall not have two sets of weights. This applies for business and is also a metaphor for us and our values. We should not have two sets of standards. One for me and one for you. We need the same values for all. If I can do it, so can others. The values I have for myself have to be the same values that I have for the other person.

As the Jews were leaving Egypt, Amalek and his warriors attacked from the rear and killed the weaker people, those people who were not able to keep up. When we go after the weakest we are searching for victims. In the animal kingdom, this is how the killing animal feeds. At the end of the parsha, we are told to never forget Amalek. This isn't just to remember a bad guy. It is to remind us never to treat people, even enemies, the way Amalek treated the Jewish people.

Yoga—Core strength

Our core values are those that guide our behavior with the external world as well as with our close relatives and friends.
We strengthen our core, the central muscles.
Lie down on ground.
Raise your legs straight up and point your toes.
Place your hands palm down on the ground next to you.
Pull your hands towards your upper body without moving them.
This is resistance pulling.
Slowly, lower your legs, using your stomach muscles.
No gritting of teeth or pulling from your neck.
When your feet touch the ground, splay them outward.

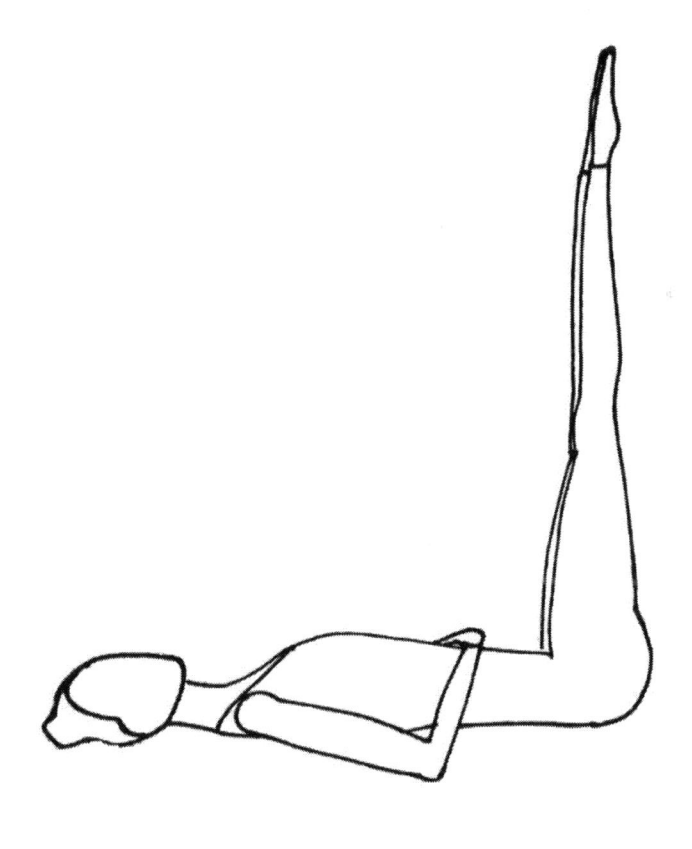

Linda Hoffman

Ki Savo (when you come in)

Parsha Insight — Blessings and curses

The people are standing on the shores of the Jordan. When you enter the land that Hashem your God gives you, show gratitude by taking the first fruits of your work and giving them to the Kohen. If you plant a tree in year one, you won't get fruit till year three or four. It is that long-awaited fruit that is to be given to the Kohen.

This parsha is always read about two weeks before Rosh Hashanah, and because Rosh Hashanah is a time of reflection on our behavior, the parsha's major theme is that we are responsible for our actions. There is cause and effect. If we fulfill Hashem's laws and do the mitzvahs properly and if we give charity, then we merit blessings. But if we did not do these things, then we are not blessed; we are cursed.

For the second time (the first being in Leviticus, parsha Bechukotal), the Torah tells us that pain and suffering that will be the Jewish people's portion for forsaking the Torah. In this parsha Moses is speaking. Read the curses: they are horrific and very hard to read. If we don't do what God says, if we don't follow the Torah, if we don't follow all the Commandments, terrible events will occur. We will eat our babies. Animals eat their young. If we don't follow Torah and Hashem's way, we will act like animals.

When these blessings and curses were spoken by Moses, they were softened by the words, "Hashem will." Hashem means Adonoy, the name of God which focuses on His mercy. Moses was putting mercy into each of the curses. If we do teshuva, if we repent, then these curses won't happen. This is the theme for Rosh Hashanah and Yom Kippur.

Why are the words from Moses so horrific? They seem to be more real coming from another human rather than from Hashem.

Think of all the problems and grief and kvetching over beef, spies, etc. Moses might have felt that since this is his last day on earth, if he doesn't get their attention now, when will he? Sometimes to get people's attention they have to be shocked.

The overall theme is that these commandments are for our benefit. They were given to us to benefit us and not to make our lives more difficult. If we choose to walk away from them, we have to realize that within the mitzvah is the benefit and within the mitzvah is the curse. Just as we said before, don't be afraid of the father warning about cars on the street, be fearful of putting ourselves in harm's way. This is Moses' last day on earth and he wants to make sure we realize the cause and effect of our behavior.

Yoga—Warnings and benefits

The blessing and the curses are very strong. How do we accept this parsha without being terrified?
Let's look at what you risk by not exercising.
Please discuss this with your personal health care provider.
Then we will look at the positive effects of regular exercise.

What can happen if we don't exercise?
Obesity.
High blood pressure.
Heart disease.
Type 2 diabetes.
Sluggish mentally and physically.
Your muscles will atrophy.
Our bones will lose density and become brittle.
We will be out of breath a lot.
Pretty horrific!

What can happen if we do exercise?
More muscle strength.
Flexibility.
Stretching.
Good balance.
Well-being.
Improved memory.
Positive force on blood pressure and heart.
Mood improvement.
Pretty great!

Thinking about caring for my health like this provides me with an understanding and ability to deal with the curses without being terrified. It is a way to take fear and turn it into a positive force. Knowing the negatives should not immobilize us, as long as we do something about them.

Nitzavim (are standing)
Vayeilech (and went)

Parsha Insight — Choose life

The parsha begins with "you are standing together, all of you, before Hashem your God." This softens all the curses from last week. It says: with all the things that went on, all the curses and blessings — look, you are still standing. With all the negative things you have done, you are still standing. Which means that Hashem (Adonoy, God's name that reflects His merciful aspect) had mercy on you and even though you did negative things, you are still standing.

A covenant is a commitment to do something and seal it in an auspicious way, such as bris mila (ritual circumcision). The covenant being made in this parsha is unique because all the other covenants are individually accepted by each person. This covenant is for all the people and means that if I'm part of all the people, my obligation to all the people is the same as my obligation to myself. So if I see someone doing something against Torah, a sin, I have an obligation to tell them that what they are doing is detrimental to themselves and to all the Jewish people. In other words, we do not let anyone else sin. In the physical center of Torah is the root of all: "Do no harm." We cannot let anyone sin. We stop them from doing harm to themselves and by extension to all the Jewish people. The people must remain united.

Now this does not mean that we run around confronting someone who we know is Jewish and we see eating a non-kosher hot dog. What it does mean is that we are part of the total community.

We are the average of our five closest associates. Choose well. If we hang around with people who do good things, it makes it easy for us to do good also. If we hang around with people who do bad things, we will eventually do what they do because we are part of that crowd. If we have a friend who goes to cocktail lounges and sits on a bar stool and talks loudly and we are with her, what she is and how she appears to others is how we appear as well. We need to protect ourselves and pick our companions wisely.

We are not responsible for hidden sins. If people are doing hidden sins, the community at large cannot be responsible for them. The only one who knows about them is God. We are responsible for members of our community—not about the person eating a non-kosher hot dog—but if we are at a board meeting, and someone proposes a bad idea, it is our responsibility to right the idea and explain why it is not appropriate. If we see wrong in something and do nothing, it perpetuates. This is where responsibility to community comes in. A good example would be a Jewish community board planning a function and discussing whether or not the food served should be kosher. It is our obligation to say that Jewish organizations must serve Jews kosher food.

Why should we not say something about the individual eating a non-kosher hot dog? The reason for this is that we should not embarrass someone. Perhaps the occasion will arise when we can quietly and privately speak to the person about kosher foods. Maybe they did not know that kosher style is not kosher.

My responsibility to the people in my community is less than the responsibility of the president of my home owners' association. The president's greater responsibility is because of position. My responsibility to the members of my shul is much less than the rabbi's because his greater position creates the greater responsibility. If I tell you I have stomach problems and you tell me that ginger ale is good for that, but my doctor told me to take this medicine, his responsibility is greater than yours. I can choose to listen to you, but you are not going to be accountable for your advice.

This whole parsha is about teshuva, going back to where we were before we sinned. We clean up our act. People wear white on Yom Kippur to symbolize their teshuva. They recognized their sin, they regretted it, they promise never to repeat it and they return to the sinless state they were in previously. They wear the white of purity and the angels.

There are obstacles to teshuva. It is hard to see ourselves. It is hard to see what we are doing wrong. If we rob a bank, we know. When we talk about someone, it is loshon hora, bad speech. We are talking because the talking is giving us pleasure. We don't see that speaking about people is bad. We think and rationalize that we are just making conversation. It is difficult to see the harm. Most of our behavior is habitual. We are used to doing something in a particular way. We don't think about it, so it doesn't occur to us to change. If we have to change, it is a lot of effort.

The parsha ends with, "Choose life." Choosing life is choosing joy, choosing peace in your relations with other people, and choosing to be happy. These are choices. Why are people unhappy? People are unhappy because they are not grateful for what they have. They are not satisfied. They are greedy and want something else, or want more. They are jealous.

We have the expectations of having it all. We are guilty of looking at other people and wanting what they have. Choosing life doesn't mean just to be healthy and stay alive: it means to choose to live each day alive with joy and peace.

At the end Moses said, "I am a hundred and twenty years old today; I can no longer go out and come in." This means that Moses has met all his goals. He had done all the things he set out to do. The only goal he had left was to go into Israel and God said he could not go.

Moses puts his affairs in order and finishes his work. He ensures an unquestioned transition of leadership to his student Joshua.

It was Joshua's turn now to lead the nation. "Be strong and courageous." Moses said this "before the eyes of all Israel." Be strong means be a leader and have humility to make it easier for people to work with you. Be courageous and stand by your convictions. When leadership is passed to someone else, the people need to know that the job is being delegated to the new person and that the person has responsibility and authority to perform. We saw this with Aaron and we see it again with Joshua.

Yoga—Come back to exercise

Since we studied teshuva, return, let us look at returning to exercise after an absence of some time. Maybe you had an injury, or you were traveling, or just got away from the routine of exercise.

Come back slowly.
Reduce the amount of time of your practice.
Perhaps do a chair exercise until you build up the strength for more rigorous exercise.
Bend your legs in your standing positions or forward bends.

If you have an injury or you have not done yoga or other exercises for a while, come back gradually so you do not hurt yourself. Be kind to your body. Don't force and create extra stress. Be sure to talk to your doctor about the type of exercise you want to do and take his advice.

Little by little, you will regain your previous strength and be able to return to your regular exercise routine.

Haazinu (give ear)
Vezos HaBerachah (and this is the blessing)

Parsha Insight — Torah is a circle

On Simchas Torah, we read the last Torah portion, Vezos HaBerachah, then proceed immediately to the first chapter of Genesis, Bereishis, reminding us that the Torah is a circle, and never ends. However, for this lesson we put Haazinu and Vezos HaBerachah together.

Haazinu is a flowing song. The whole parsha is a song. It is the past, present and future and back and forth. Everything is one big circle and everything is united. The beginning of the parsha, "Give ear, O **heavens**, and I will speak; and may the **earth** hear the words of my mouth. May my teaching drop like **rain**, may my utterance flow like the **dew**; like storm **winds** upon **vegetation**..."

Take these words and go back to Bereishis, and let's see the very first posik: "In the beginning of God's creating the **heavens** and the **earth**— when the earth was astonishingly empty, with darkness upon the surface of the deep, and the Divine Presence hovered upon the surface of the waters— Let there be a **firmament** in the midst of the waters..." Firmament usually refers to atmosphere and it is separating the **upper waters** (clouds, rain) from the **lower waters** (oceans or dew). The **winds** may be the firmament. "God called the dry land Earth...Let the earth sprout **vegetation**..."

The beginning of Haazinu is the beginning of Bereishis, although it is written differently. Haazinu alludes to the past, present and future in this way throughout the parsha. This is why the name is Haazinu, give ear. Listen, and listen with thought. Hear the message and consider the words as a complete allusion to the story of the Jews. This is a review of the history, of the whole Torah. The 613 words in Haazinu represent the 613 mitzvahs. Each word is said to allude to a mitzvah.

Ramban said that everything is in this song. It refers to all of Torah and takes us through history to the present and on to the future.

Moses said, "May my teachings be like rain." Rain drops from the sky, and it helps things grow. Rain is indiscriminating. When it drops and waters the ground, it helps both plants and weeds. God's teachings drop like rain and assist the good and the bad. Being imperfect humans, we need to improve our middos and have good character. These teachings will enable the good middos to grow and enhance us and help us achieve our greatest potential.

The teachings, when falling on bad middos, can be used as rationalizations, excuses and complaints, and then all they are doing is shoring up negative behavior. Knowledge of a subject can be used for good or bad. We have to be vigilant. Those with evil intent will take the teachings and convert them to evil.

All of history is on a continuum, in the days of yore, and the years of every generation. We look at the broad aspect of 6000 years or the much narrower picture of our own lives. The history of me at twenty formed the base for me at forty, and the lessons of each stage of my life bring me to the present and will be the template for my future. Everything that happens in the past goes forward and creates the future. I love to look at the Purim story and see how the entire tale played out over some thirteen years. The pieces fell into place just as God, the King (when the Purim story says the king, it refers to God), wanted them to occur.

When we study Torah we see how one parsha leads into the next parsha. We see how a theme repeats itself. Consider the children of the Avos. Abraham had Ishmael and Isaac and only Isaac was fit to create the offspring for the Jewish people. Isaac's sons were Esau and Jacob and only Jacob created the twelve tribes of Israel. Adam's son, Cain, after killing Abel, did not form the lineage of the Jews. Adam's lineage flowed from Seth. Noah's lineage came from Shem and not his firstborn, Japheth. There is nothing new in history.

In our own lives we see the same thing. We keep repeating the same patterns over and over again. We are trying and trying and hoping — now I'll get it right. Sometimes we open our eyes, open our ears, and we see that there is a different way. We get it! And we change. Sometimes it takes a crisis. Sometimes Hashem changes everything in our lives, and then we understand.

The holidays of Rosh Hashanah and Yom Kippur are for us to open our eyes and take a really good look. We see the error of our ways. Are we going to make some changes? What are we going to do? What is our action plan?

Hashem told Moses to climb Mount Nevo and look across at Israel. Moses cannot go into Israel; he will die on the mountain.

Vezos HaBerachah is a bracha, a blessing for the twelve tribes. "And this is the blessing of Moses, the Man of God." This is the first time in all of Torah that Moses is called the Man of God. Moses blesses the Children of Israel according to the tribes, just as Jacob blessed each of his sons. Moses gives a blessing that applies to their characteristics and history, and this is what Jacob did when he blessed his sons on his deathbed. Each son and each tribe has a different blessing dependent upon their individual middos. This is the circular pattern of Torah. The entire Torah circles and repeats. Jacob blessing his sons is repeated in Moses blessing the Children of Israel, his children.

The parsha ends with, "Never again has there arisen in Israel a prophet like Moses, whom Hashem had known face to face."

In shul on the festival of Simchas Torah, this parsha is read and then the Torah is rolled forward to the first parsha. The reading continues with Bereishis, "In the beginning of God's creating..." Such a powerful moment. On Simchas Torah, many shuls give every post-bar mitzvah male present the opportunity to be called to the Torah. The sedra (reading the last posik in Vezos HaBerachah and the first posik in Bereishis) is read repeatedly until everyone has received an aliyah.

We have finished our study of Torah. We celebrate with a siyum—a celebration marking the completion of any unit of Torah study, or book of the Mishnah or Talmud in Judaism. A siyum is usually followed by a celebratory meal, or seudat mitzvah, a meal in honor of a mitzvah, or commandment.

Please, be sure to celebrate the cycle of the completion of the Torah reading. Thank you for letting me share with you and may this be the start of many future, healthy years of Torah study. The Torah is not a distant thing. It is always with us and always available.

Yoga—Basic seated pose

Seated on floor cross-legged.
Palms up on knees.
Ready to receive.

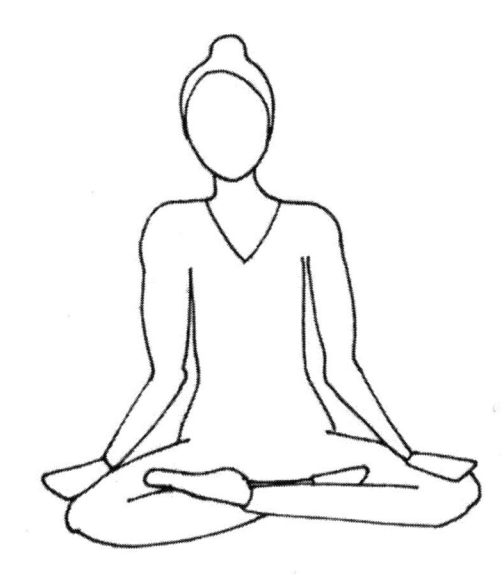

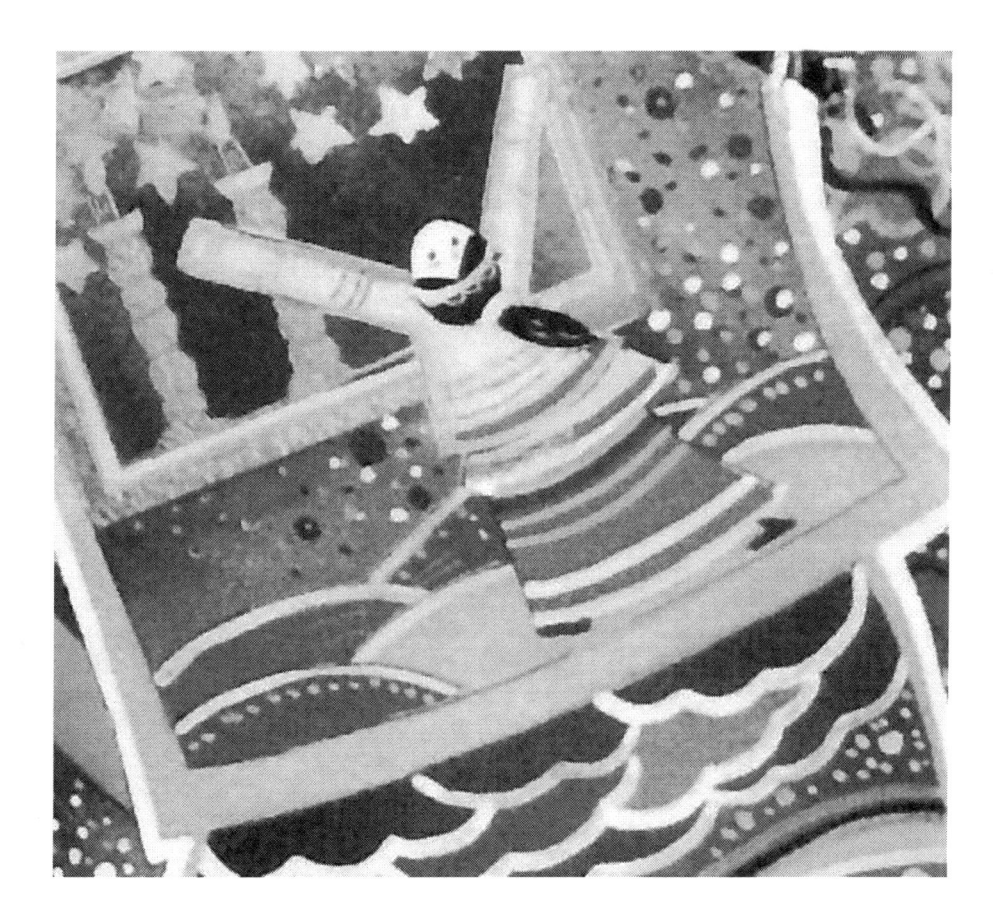

References

References

Torah Leaders Referenced

Rabbeinu Bachya, Bahya ben Joseph ibn Paquda, 11th century, Spain, *Guide to the Duties of the Heart*

Chazon Ish, Avrohom Yeshaya Karelitz (1878-1953)

Chofetz Chaim, Rabbi Yisrael Meir Kagan HaKohen, 1838-1933, Radun, Poland,
Guard Your Tongue (loshon hora), *Mishnah Berurah, Shulchan Aruch*

Rabbi Samson Raphael Hirsch, the laws of purity, commentary on the Torah

Rabbi Shlomo Luntschitz 1550-1619, Torah commentary Kli Yakar

Rambam, Maimonides, Rabbi Moshe ben Maimon, 1135-1204, Spain, Morocco, known for systematic code of Halachah, Mishneh Torah, *The Guide to the Perplexed*; physician and philosopher

Ramban, Nachmanides, Rabbi Moshe ben Nachman, 1194-1270, Catalonia, Spain; known for Torah commentary that incorporates Kabbalah

Rashi, Rabbi Shlomo ben Yitzchak, 1040-1105, Troyes, France; known for p'shat or simple meaning of Torah

Rabbi Yisroel Salanter, 1810-1883, Konigsberg, was the father of the Musar movement in Orthodox Judaism and a famed rosh yeshiva and Talmudist

Rabbi Mendel Weinbach, co-founder and dean of Ohr Somayach, 1933-2012, was an Orthodox Jewish rabbi and one of the fathers of the modern-day baal teshuva

Rabbi Noah Weinberg, Aish.com, was an Orthodox Jewish rabbi, rosh yeshiva, and a father of today's baal teshuva

Books

Awesome Creation, Rabbi Yosef Bitton, Gefen Publishing House
Beloved Companions, Rabbi Yisroe Pesach Feinhandler
Bible Basics, Jerome S. Hahn, International Traditions Corp.
Chofetz Chaim, A Daily Companion, Mesorah Publications
The Chumash, The Stone Edition, ArtScroll Series
Daily Dose of Torah, ArtScroll Series, 14 volumes, Kleinman Edition
The Garden of Emuna, Rabbi Shalom Arush
Gateway to Judaism, Rabbi Mordechai Becher, Shaar Press Publication
The Gemstones in the Breastplate, E. Raymond Capt, Artisan Publishers
Genesis and the Big Bang, Gerald Lawrence Schroeder, Bantam 1990
Growth Through Torah, Rabbi Zelig Pliskin, Bnay Yakov Publications
Guide to the Perplexed-The Mitzvos, Part III, Rambam
Living Each Week, Rabbi Abraham J. Twerski, ArtScroll Series
Middos, Rebbetzin S. Feldbrand, Lishmoa Lilmod U'Lelamed Publisher
The Midrash Says, Rabbi Moshe Weissman, Bnay Yakov Publications, five volumes
Psychotherapy and Prayer, Dr. Jeffrey M. Last, Feldheim Publishers
Sayings of the Fathers, Pirkei Avos, Behrman House, Rabbi Joseph H. Hertz
Unlocking the Torah Text, Rabbi Shmuel Golden, Gefen Publishing House, four volumes
Values, Prosperity and the Talmud, Larry Kahaner, John Wiley & Sons, Inc.

Internet Research

Judaism.about.com
Aish.com
Azamra.com
chabad.org
kesertorah.org
learning-styles-online.com
MatsMatsMats.com
www.mayoclinic.com
Ohr.edu
torah.org
yashanet.com
www.wikipedia.org

Made in the USA
Coppell, TX
28 May 2020